Cerebral Palsy

MERLIN J. MECHAM

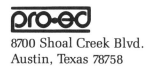

8700 Shoal Creek Blvd.
Austin, Texas 78758

The PRO-ED
studies in
communicative disorders

Series editor
HARVEY HALPERN

Library of Congress Cataloging in Publication Data
Mecham, Merlin J.
  Cerebral palsy.

  (The Pro-Ed studies in communicative disorders)
  Bibliography: p.
    1. Cerebral palsy—Complications and sequelae. 2. Communicative
disorders. 3. Cerebral palsied children.
I. Title. II. Series. [DNLM. 1. Cerebral Palsy. WS 342 M486c]
RC388.M39   1986   618.92'836   86-3271
ISBN 0-89079-087-6

8700 Shoal Creek Blvd.
Austin, Texas 78758

          10 9 8 7 6 5 4 3 2   89 90 91

Contents

Preface

This monograph provides an up-to-date and concise discussion of cerebral palsy. The first section gives a general description of the group of syndromes found in this condition as well as the medical, social, and educational implications. The second section suggests the role of the multidimensional team of professionals ordinarily required to deal with the cerebral palsied child. It summarizes Public Law 94-142 and the impact of this legislation on resources for severely handicapped children at various age levels. The third section presents the communication problems commonly encountered and their neurolinguistic and dysarthric concomitants. The fourth section discusses assessment, and a fifth section describes treatment approaches that have been found effective, including neurodevelopmental, physiological, and compensatory approaches.

Cerebral Palsy

Cerebral Palsy and Its Implications

Cerebral palsy is a nonprogressive neuromuscular disorder caused by damage to the immature higher brain centers; the brain is considered mature at 16 years of age (Batshaw & Perret, 1981).

Cerebral means brain-centered, and *palsy* means lack of muscle control. Older terms for the condition proved to be unsatisfactory. Little's disease, a term reflecting the name of the British physician who first described the condition, was a 19th-century label. Spasticity, a term describing a specific type of cerebral palsy, was used in the early years of the 20th century. The term cerebral palsy (CP) was suggested by Dr. W. Phelps (1950), an orthopedic surgen, to more nearly describe a cluster of differing symptomotologies that would differentiate this syndrome from polio, which was in a peak epidemic at that time. The nonprogressive characteristic of the syndrome means that the victim does not get worse as time goes on.

Factors causing cerebral palsy are generally divided into three categories: prenatal, paranatal (during birth), and postnatal. This temporal division was suggested by Hayman in 1938 and has been popular since (Courville, 1954). A fairly large percentage (about 40%) of cerebral palsy occurrences are from unknown causes. Known causes include insult during the first trimester as a result of radiation exposure, intrauterine infection, ingestion of teratogenic drugs, or chromosomal abnormalities; damage in later stages of pregnancy resulting from such things as abruptio placenta (premature detachment); birth complica-

1

tions during labor and delivery; and neonatal complications such as prematurity, asphyxia, and sepsis (toxoplasmosis) (Batshaw & Perret, 1981, p. 193).

Orthopedic classifications in cerebral palsy describe visible neuromuscular symptoms. These descriptions include place or location—monoplegia (one extremity), hemiplegia (two homolateral extremities), paraplegia (the two lower extremities), triplegia (three extremities), and quadriplegia (four extremities); type of involvement—spasticity, athetosis, ataxia, tremor, rigidity; and severity—mild, moderate, severe, or profound.

Various combinations of place, type, and severity may occur in any given child. Types of cerebral palsy are further defined in neurological terms describing the neurological systems most affected. Pyramidal lesions generally result in spasticity (about 50% of the total group), while extrapyramidal lesions generally result in athetosis and/or tremor (see Figure 1).

Correlation of orthopedic and neurological classifications results in a system of classification that has often been used because it gives general and combined understanding of the complex matrix of cerebral palsy conditions.

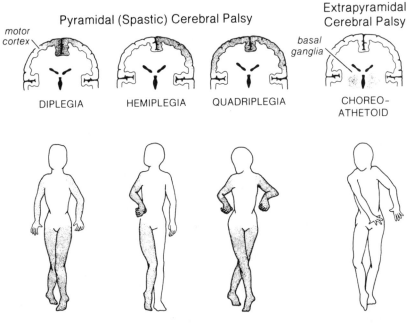

Figure 1. The various forms of cerebral palsy and the regions of the brain affected. From Batshaw and Perret (1981, p. 195). Drawing by Elaine Kasmer. Copyright 1981 by Mark L. Batshaw and Yvonne M. Perret. Reprinted by permission.

Mixed types of cerebral palsy occur quite frequently (about 25% of the total group); a mixed CP condition may have predominantly spastic muscle involvement and secondarily athetotic muscular involvement, or just the reverse, depending on whether the major lesion is primarily in the pyramidal or extrapyramidal system. Since brain damage in mixed types is usually extensive, "these children are usually mentally retarded and have other associated disabilities" (Batshaw & Perret, 1981, p. 196).

Diagnostically, one of the major signs of cerebral palsy in infancy is the persistence of primitive reflexes (Capute et al., 1977), which can be identified through manifestation of particular reflexive patterns unique to each type of reflex; such reflexes usually interfere with proper and timely development in sitting, head balance, rolling over, and creeping and crawling in early infancy. The most common primative reflexes to persist in cerebral palsy are the asymmetrical tonic neck reflexes (ATNR), the tonic labyrinthine reflexes (TLR), and the positive support reflex (PSR) (Batshaw & Perret, 1981). Each is illustrated in Figures 2, 3, and 4, respectively.

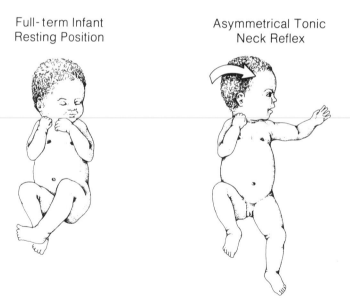

Full-term Infant
Resting Position

Asymmetrical Tonic
Neck Reflex

Figure 2. The asymmetrical tonic neck reflex, or fenser's response. As the head is turned, the arm and leg on the same side as the chin extend, and the other arm and leg flex. From Batshaw and Perret (1981, p. 196). Drawing by Elaine Kasmer. Copyright 1981 by Mark L. Batshaw and Yvonne M. Perret. Reprinted by permission.

Tonic Labyrinthine Reflex

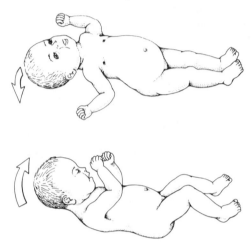

Figure 3. The tonic labyrinthine reflex. Extension of the head backward leads to retraction of the shoulders and extension of the legs. From Batshaw and Perret (1981, p. 197). Drawing by Elaine Kasmer. Copyright 1981 by Mark L. Batshaw and Yvonne M. Perret. Reprinted by permission.

Positive Support Reflex

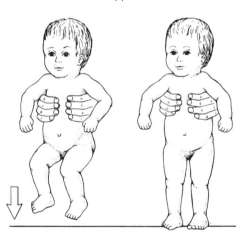

Figure 4. The positive support reflex. As the baby is bounced, the legs straighten to support the baby's weight. From Batshaw and Perret (1981, p. 198). Drawing by Elaine Kasmer. Copyright 1981 by Mark L. Batshaw and Yvonne M. Perret. Reprinted by permission.

During early childhood and the preschool years, the most obvious deficits among cerebral palsied children are ones affecting mobility and self-help. The most devastating is quadriplegic involvement, the least devastating is hemiplegia, while somewhere in between fall the conditions of triplegia and paraplegia (Batshaw & Perret, 1981).

Approximately 60% of individuals with cerebral palsy have some degree of mental retardation (Hohman & Freedheim, 1958). About 35% are plagued with seizures at some time during their lives (Batshaw & Perret, 1981).

Incidence and Prognosis

Various studies of the incidence of cerebral palsy have varied slightly (Mecham, Berko, & Berko, 1960), but most suggest that there are approximately 6 CPs born in every 1,000 live births in the United States. With modern, improved technologies in prenatal and paranatal care, as well as improved diagnostic procedures, it is probable that the incidence of CP has diminished during the past few years (Batshaw & Perret, 1981; United Cerebral Palsy Telethon, 1984). Life expectancy is somewhat less than for the average population; about 10% become solely self-supporting, about 40% are employed in sheltered workshops, 36% are partially independent at home, and about 15% are mostly dependent upon others for their care and well-being (O'Reilly, 1975).

Medical Implications

Although physical, occupational, and speech therapies are often under the prescriptive supervision of the medical practitioner, the major contributions of medicine fall mainly in the areas of drugs, neurolytic procedures, surgery, and braces.

Drugs have been used for relaxation with varying degrees of success. Sedatives such as phenobarbital, narcotics, and bromides were used in the early days, but they are not now felt to be very helpful because they make the patient drowsy and listless. Currently the two most commonly used medications are Valium and Dantrium (Batshaw & Perret, 1981). Valium tones down the central nervous system and thus effects relaxation of the muscles indirectly. Dantrium "reduces spasticity by acting directly on the muscle fibers and neuromuscular junction" (Batshaw & Perret, 1981, p. 204). Only about half of the children who were researched with this drug showed improvement, and this turned out to be very modest. The undesirable side effects often make the decision to use drugs somewhat tenuous.

Neurolytic procedures involve the blocking of nerve impulses in the stretch reflex arc by injecting such chemicals as phenol or alcohol at the point where the nerves enter the muscles (intramuscular neurolysis) (Easton & Halpern, 1981, p. 149).

Two types of surgery—orthopedic and neurosurgery—have been used with severe cases of muscular contractions or deformities (Batshaw & Perret, 1981). Orthopedic surgery is performed to disconnect, lengthen, or transfer affected muscles. Neurosurgery has generally been found to be less satisfactory (Batshaw & Perret, 1981). It has ranged from ventrolateral thalamotomy to placing an electrode stimulator in certain parts of the central nervous system.

At this time, the most useful approach to medical treatment lies in the area of bracing and special seating equipment. Braces have been found useful in cerebral palsy to control involuntary movements, prevent contractures, and provide needed stabilization for sitting, standing, and walking. Braces range in size from short ankle splints to full-length braces that extend from the ankles up to the hips and, in rare cases, to the top of the head. Most braces are made of molded plastic. Since they are custom-made, they are changed as the child grows. The use of these devices "may improve functioning, decrease the risk of contractures, and prevent or delay the need for corrective orthopedic surgery" (Batshaw & Perret, 1981, p. 204).

A large number of children with severe cerebral palsy are nonambulatory and thus rely upon wheelchairs for mobility. A modified wheelchair not only gives the child unlimited mobility but also provides good support for proper posturing. Figure 5 illustrates a chair without the use of special posturing inserts and restrainers; Figure 6 illustrates a chair after inserts and restrainers are properly in place.

Behavioral and Social Implications

Perceptual, emotional, and adaptive deficits provide obstacles to behavioral-social adjustment ranging all the way from slight to severe.

The educational implications of the perceptual disturbances of the cerebral palsied child have been elaborated by Cruickshank and Bice (1955) and Cruickshank and Dolphin (1951). Perhaps the most frequently mentioned perceptual disturbance is hyperirritable attention (Berko, Berko, & Thompson, 1970). A child with hyperirritable attention is unable to refrain from reacting to various stimuli in the environment. The resulting symptoms are short attention span, hyperactivity or restlessness, impulsivity, and sometimes vacillating attention.

Other perceptual problems that may make learning difficult for the CP child include perceptual rigidity (desire to have environmental contexts and schedules the same all the time), dissociation (inability to synthesize aspects of a situation into a meaningful Gestalt), disinhition (manipulating objects in stereotyped and more or less random fashion), and difficulty in figure-ground organization.

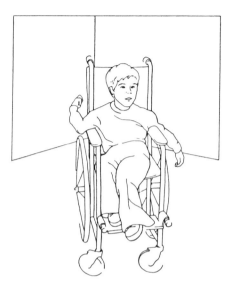

Figure 5. Child's position in wheelchair prior to use of inserts. From McDonald (1976, p. 110). Copyright 1976 by PRO-ED. Reprinted by permission.

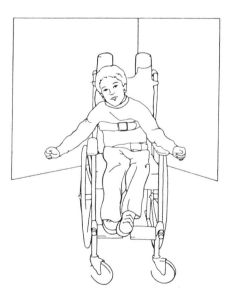

Figure 6. Positioning of child with inserts in place. From McDonald (1976, p. 110). Copyright 1976 by PRO-ED. Reprinted by permission.

Difficulties in initiating movements and in organizing the perceptual field may cause what has been termed by Berko, Berko, and Thompson (1970) *initiatory delay and confusion.* In this situation the child often takes an inordinate amount of time to respond to a particular request or question. One may erroneously misinterpret this as lack of comprehension when in reality the child has comprehended and merely needs time to organize a proper response; often this takes as much as 40 seconds (Berko, Berko, & Thompson, 1970, p. 44).

Two types of emotional problems in cerebral palsy are described in the literature: emotional lability (which is an autonomic nervous system hyperexcitatory response comprised of flushing, incongruous laughing, palling, gagging, etc.) and emotional upsets (which stem primarily from the environment). Glick (1953a) sureyed 200 cerebral palsied adults selected from case loads of two social agencies in New York City. These cerebral palsied adults were ambulatory and between the ages of 18 and 45. Three fourths of this group reported indications of emotional maladjustment. The emotional instability of 20% was serious enough to preclude the possibilities of job placement. Various types of problems appeared to be quite salient: unrealistic attitudes (42%), excessive fears (51%), and lack of motivation (70%). Instability was reported more frequently in cases having mild physical handicaps.

Glick (1953a) found that only 21% of the 200 adults she studied were employed. The main sources of problems in employment included limitations resulting from physical, mental, and emotional problems, inadequate vocational guidance and preparation for job placement, and resistance of employers to hiring the cerebral palsied due to lack of understanding or prejudice or fear on the part of employers. Problems found by these older studies appear to be still prevalent, perhaps to a slightly reduced extent (Easton & Halpern, 1981).

One would be hard put to talk about adaptive problems without mentioning the impact that communication problems may have. It is quite well known that cerebral palsied individuals are almost always plagued with communicative disabilities ranging all the way from relatively mild and noninterfering to profound to the point of being completely unintelligible and/or nonvocal. Communication problems and their impact on adaptiveness are discussed in greater detail in a later section.

Educational Implications

When one considers that education still entails the mastery of the three R's, most of which depend upon spoken and/or written communication for their mastery, it behooves us to look at the vehicles for spoken and written communication available to the cerebral palsied child. The most important conventional vehicles for mastery of the three R's are the eye (for visual communication, or reading); the ear (for auditory communication, or listening); the arm and hand (for graphic communication, or writing); and the voice and articulation (for vocal communication, or speaking). When we look at the incidence and severity of involvement of these various aspects of communication, we find the cerebral palsied child at a considerable disadvantage. Estimates have it that 40% of cerebral palsied children have defective vision (Batshaw & Perret, 1981), 13.3% have impaired hearing, 78.5% have arm and/or hand involvement on the right side, and 70–80% have moderate to profound vocal-communication problems (Hopkins, Brice, & Colton, 1954). These estimates, coupled with the other known perceptual, emotional, adaptive, and intellectual problems, begin to give us some notion of why a large proportion of the cerebral palsied population is classified as severely handicapped educationally and in need of a multidisciplinary and very special educational curriculum.

Since needs begin so early and continue over practically a whole lifetime, there is a need for a continuum of resources and support systems in every community.

Continuum of Resources

The final common pathway in both the long-term and short-term planning should be programming based upon the joint thinking of various professional team members. In addition, special programs should be available for the child at various age levels – infant and toddler years, preschool years, early school years, and social-vocational adjustment. The nature and functions of the interdisciplinary team and the impact of PL 94-142 upon the development and implementation of special programs for the severely handicapped are discussed in greater detail in the next section.

Multidimensional and Team Approach to Treatment

Public Law 94-142 and Its Impact

Possibly the two most important aspects of PL 94-142 are its stress on the importance of the individual (developmental/educational) plan for each child and the necessity of an interdisciplinary team approach.

Individual development/educational plans for severely cerebral palsied children might more appropriately be called the "individual life plan" (ILP), since it must of necessity span the entire life of those individuals who will be highly dependent upon special resources and significant others to achieve the most optimal and rewarding adaptive life. These plans, by their nature, must be planned individually for each person and are likely to differ significantly from one person to another because of the great heterogeneity of strengths and/or deficits to be found within this particular syndrome. Furthermore, an ILP changes significantly as the individual grows older and as capabilities expand.

In spite of these considerable differences, the plans for all persons include some common domains and also require input and interaction from a nucleus of professions.

The domains common to all ILPs include perceptual-motor skills, social skills, communicative skills, and adaptive-vocational skills. Some of these domains have greatest importance in the early years, while others may be more important as the child gets older. Some domains may be very strong modalities for a given child, while others may be difficult or impossible to achieve. Some domains will require the participation of all important team members, while some require the participation of only one or two.

The interdisciplinary team members needed to develop and help implement the ILP includes parents, physical therapist, occupational therapist, classroom teacher, psychologist, physician, nurse, school administrator, speech-language pathologist, and audiologist (Mecham, Berko, & Berko, 1960). The importance and role of each team member depends upon the priorities and curriculum included in each ILP. Some members of the interdisciplinary team become more important or play a more predominant role at certain ages (or in certain domains) than others. The parent's role, for example, requires maximum involvement, more so than any other team member during the infant, toddler, and preschool years.

The individual life plan of all cerebral palsied children is commonly divided into developmental life-age phases in terms of various resources that are promoted through public law for different-aged children. These life-age phases divide quite naturally into (1) infant and toddler years, (2) preschool years, (3) early school years, and (4) later school and early adult years. The legal ages covered by PL 94-142, for example, are kindergarten through age 21 by mandate and 0 through 5 for schools that include programs for normal children anywhere within that age bracket. The following discussion will cover the domains, personnel, and resources available to children at these various life-phases of the ILP.

Infant and Toddler Years

During the infant and toddler stage (0 through 24 months) the most important domains in the ILP are care for the child's personal needs and sensorimotor development as outlined by Piaget. Personal-care needs include feeding, dressing, bathing and cleaning, carrying, and health maintenance. The sensorimotor development includes ambulation, fine-motor skills, vision, hearing, and so forth. Normal scales of development are useful if their milestones have a high degree of ordinal consistency (consistent order of emergency across children). High ordinal consistency (90% or more) provides the best index boundaries of sensitivity periods within which development of specific milestones seems to have the greatest degree of efficiency. The sensorimotor modules described by Uzgiris and Hunt (1975) have been shown to have within them a high degree of ordinal consistency of the various milestones; therefore, they provide an excellent basis for setting up objectives at a time when sensitivity for their acquisition would be maximal.

Since cerebral palsied children vary greatly in their rate of acquisition, the order of milestones to be included in the curriculum is a much better index for setting up objectives than the child's chronological age. Two children who are the same age may differ greatly in rate of acquisition (one child may develop a milestone at 10 months and the other at 30 months), but the order in which they develop the particular milestone relative to other milestones is approximately the same. This principle enables one to use *order* as an indication of when to encourage development of particular milestones (if ordinal consistency of the various milestones included in the ILP is high). Ordinal consistency of various sensorimotor milestones included in the Uzgiris and Hunt (1975) scales ranged from 95% to 100%.

Persons carrying the primary role in personal care and sensorimotor development during the infant/toddler stage are the parents and the family physician. Other specialists with important roles during this stage include the neurologist, orthopedist, speech pathologist, psychologist, and audiologist. These latter specialists are usually available for special consultations with the parents and family physician.

Special resource programs outside of the home for children this young are rare, and usually available only to more severely handicapped children. Parents must carry the major burden of care and training for children at this age. The only major resource other than the home, either natural or adopted, is a special institution for the mentally retarded and physically handicapped. The tendency for early institutionalization has greatly diminished since the advent of PL 94-142. As a rule, resources in the community and outside the institution are much more enriching and profitable for the children. Parents can anticipate entering their child into a special program at the preschool and/or early school level, and therefore are faced with the challenge of getting the child as ready as possible for entrance into those programs.

During the infant/toddler stage, there are a number of health problems that frequently occur and may need attention. These include contractures, bowel and bladder incontinence, constipation, osteoporosis, degenerative joint problems, malnutrition, respiratory infections, seizures, fatigue, and others. It is usually important to try to determine whether the child may have any visual or hearing deficits.

Parents often seem overwhelmed when faced with the special care required by a severely physically handicapped child and are often at a loss in knowing how to cope. An excellent resource for information on how parents can care for their young cerebral palsied child in the home is a book written by Nancie Finnie (1968) on this topic. Some very important areas covered in this book include feeding techniques as well as carrying and posturing procedures that minimize the occurrence of abnormal motor reflexes that interfere with behaviors requiring conscious motor or muscular control. It also suggests equipment and activities that parents may use to facilitate development of sensorimotor skills. (Of course, this book is only one kind of resource for parents and cannot serve as a substitute for professional assistance.)

Preschool Years

During the preschool years (considered mainly to be 2 through 4 years in chronological age), the most important domains in the ILP are self-help skills such as self-feeding, self-dressing, self-direction, and beginning self-cleanliness skills like washing and wiping hands, toilet training, and so on. Also important during these years is the development of Piagetian preoperational cognitive skills.

It must be again emphasized here, especially for cerebral palsied children, that chronological age is not an accurate indication of these various stages of development; some children develop rapidly, while others may develop very slowly in some skill areas but more rapidly in skill areas requiring little motor activity. Children with severe perceptual-motor deficits may develop very slowly in a wide spectrum of skills.

The most important principle for planning and monitoring a child's ILP curriculm is the principle of ordinal consistency of curricular items; milestones with high ordinal consistency serve as the best indices of the end of one readiness stage and the beginning of the other. Lack of progress in one milestone over a rather long period suggests that the particular milestone may not be productive for this child, perhaps due to specific impeding deficits, and that another milestone may be more productive.

Persons who carry a primary role in intervention with the cerebral palsied child during the preschool years are the parents and the preschool teacher—if the child is enrolled in a preschool or daytime developmental disabilities program. Enrollment in a preschool program geared to the needs of the cerebral palsied child is an optimal condition for the preschool child. A much more important role begins to emerge for the physical and occupational therapists and the speech/language pathologist; most preschools for orthopedic-deficit children have all the above specialists as either full-time or part-time staff members. In addition, medical and psychological consultations are important adjuncts. Thus we can see that the interdisciplinary team members who will interact in the development and implementation of the ILP for the preschool years is comprised of a larger number of professionals working in close coordination with the parent and teacher.

Most communities across the country now have some facilities for orthopedically handicapped preschool children; the program is likely to be part of an outpatient clinic of a children's hospital or a program made available through the state developmental disabilities program. State health departments also often have outpatient clinics with limited treatment follow-up facilities. Parents and professionals can find out what is available near a given child's residence by contacting the state social services division, the state health department, or the state or community developmental disabilities program.

The most important health-related problems that will likely need special medical attention are complications resulting from severe neuromuscular disorders or/and seizures. Bracing and/or therapy to prevent neuromuscular contractures or muscular atrophy are most important for children with severe physical involvement. Special seating and ambulation arrangements are of importance during the day both in the preschool and in the home.

The individual life plan (ILP) may be called by some other term in some preschool programs, depending upon the prevailing administrative philosophy; it may be called the individual education plan (IEP) or the individual development plan (IDP). Regardless of the label, the function is still the same: to provide an individualized plan of evaluation and intervention for each child based upon her or his particular needs. It is now the right of every child to have such a plan, to be approved and signed by the parent or guardian.

Therapeutic intervention, as physical therapy, occupational therapy, or speech/language therapy, must of course be determined by the appropriate specialists in consultation with the parent and teacher in accordance with the particular needs of the child; such therapeutic programs cannot be guided by a prepared curriculum guide. Even cognitive training, taken from some curriculum guide, must be very selective and include those objectives that the child both needs and is likely to be able to achieve in the presence of specific weaknesses or deficits. Each child has the right to the opportunity to demonstrate whether he or she can benefit from particular objectives; given optimal conditions for intervention responsiveness, the actual progress of the child should be a more important factor for omitting important goals than another person's preconceived judgments. The preplanned inclusion of important goals, however, should lean heavily upon the professional judgment of the team in selecting that combination of objectives that are both important and feasible for the child to develop at the present time. Placing goals in order of estimated difficulty allows one to select easy goals with which to begin and thus provide both motivation and success. All goals selected, utilized, and monitored must be based primarily upon the child's needs, responsivity, and motivation and only secondarily upon their presence in a published curriculum guide. Such orientation allows the team to combine the needs of the child with available resources and still maintain the integrity of the ILP.

The preschool years are the most critical period for the development of the primary language repertoire. A general guide utilizing normal language sequences tends to be very useful for children who likely have the potential for developing intelligible vocal language (see Mecham & Jones, 1981, for example). For children who will not respond to efforts in vocal language, nonvocal language symbols should still be encouraged and/or taught. A more detailed discussion of language intervention, both vocal and nonvocal, is presented in a later section.

Occupational therapy (usually in conjunction with speech therapy) plays a primary role during preschool years in helping the parent and teacher develop and carry out special training in feeding and self-help, dressing, and grooming. Physical therapy has broadened during the past 10 years to include more than just muscle-exercise training; it now includes special reflex-inhibiting postures, relaxation chairs, scooter-type bellyboards for ambulation, as well as special standing, sitting, and walking devices, which all aid the development of muscular control.

Early School Years

Early school years are usually the time when the three R's are taught as the mainstream of the educational process. Children with cerebral palsy may be able to experience graduated degrees of mainstreaming (i.e., integration into the regular classroom with normal children), depending upon the severity of their handicapping conditions and the degree to which they are able to acquire competitive academic skills.

The person most likely to play a major role in coordinating the IEP will be the school district's coordinator of special education working in conjunction with the child's parent and school principal. Most school districts typically have self-contained special education classes as well as support services such as physical therapy and speech and/or hearing therapy as needed. Children who are partially mainstreamed (i.e., integrated into the normal classroom for selected subject matter) will use the resource room or self-contained special education class as a home base and will be mainstreamed at various times during the day. Many of the severely handicapped children may not be able to be mainstreamed in any of the school curriculum and therefore will depend entirely upon the self-contained classroom for their education.

Since the curriculum for any given cerebral palsied child will be tailored to fit specific needs, it is difficult to talk about curriculum in general terms. The IEP will determine what the child will be getting during the early school years.

Members of the team participating in the development and implementation of the IEP, in addition to key persons such as the parent (or guardian), teacher, and school principal, will be professionals from the following various specialties as needed: physical therapy, occupational therapy, orthopedics, ophthalmology, psychology, social work, speech/language pathology, and audiology.

Special equipment is usually required for the more severe physical handicaps, such as relaxation chairs, specially adapted desks, communication boards, standing tables or boards, special ambulation equipment, and stabilizing braces. Again, needs for such specialized equipment will be determined by team planning and must be included in the IEP. Special schedules for individualized training, mainstreaming, and other components of the program are usually worked out by the child's home teacher.

Parents play a crucial role in the early educational planning of the cerebral palsied child; they must be involved in the development of the IEP and must approve it before it can be implemented. Parents are also involved in any changes in the IEP.

Most states have special education programs for severely handicapped children under the provisions of PL 94-142. This law provides that all children must receive an appropriate and free public education program. As a result, all school districts have an opportunity to apply for special education resources and funding in order to provide a free and appropriate education to all handicapped children within its boundaries. Many smaller districts may find it more effective to combine their resources, especially in rural areas where various specialties are less accessible.

Parents and/or specialists who wish to know more about the provision of special educational resources in their district can obtain the information from the district administrative office; if necessary, further information can be obtained from state departments of education, the U.S. Bureau of the Handicapped, and the National Council for Exceptional Children.

Late School and Early Adult Years

The late school and early adult years span the period from the mid-teens through 25 to 30 years of age. Important domains to be considered for intervention are highly variable from one individual to another. However, certain prerequisites for vocational intervention have been roughly established (Easton & Halpern, 1981). Adult prevocational and vocational potential is affected by interactions of such deficits as "joint movement and muscle strength; perceptual function; cognitive and intellectual function; memory function; attention and response abilities; and personal and social attitudes and skills" (p. 114). Efforts toward minimizing the effects of such deficits on physical independence and vocational function should be incorporated in the ILP of cerebral palsied persons during this period. Fortunately "training and provisions of assistance by aides and/or mechanical and electronic devices can improve the cerebral palsy patient's function level" (p. 144).

One of the major problems for the person with a moderately severe or severe motor disability is ambulation. Most hemiplegics will be ambulatory, as are many paraplegics; however, more severe paraplegics or quadriplegics will have serious ambulation problems. Diplegics will generally be ambulatory but may lack many of the self-help skills such as self-feeding and self-dressing.

Independent feeding and dressing are usually in the repertoire of mildly and moderately involved persons, regardless of type of cerebral palsy. Moderately involved persons may need more time to feed and dress, but can do so if given enough time. Independent feeding and dressing may be severely impaired or impossible for severely handicapped persons. Persons with contractures, especially in the shoulders, knees, or hips, may have great difficulty dressing; the presence of exaggerated reflexes (oral and/or body) may exacerbate problems in eating and dressing. Whether an inability to function independently in these skills will affect vocational training or employment is to a great extent determined by the nature of the job for which the person will be engaged. The kinds of jobs possible for the severely handicapped person are relatively few.

Another domain that may affect life adaptation of the cerebral palsied person during this period is that of personal hygiene. A severely involved person may still become fairly independent in bathing and grooming with specialized training and use of certain specialized equipment and/or modifications of the bathing facility (Easton & Halpern, 1981).

Certain psychosocial disabilities may present interference with effective vocational habilitation. As Easton and Halpern (1981) note, "personality assessment to identify the patient's behavior patterns, personal attitudes, problem-solving strategies, and level of self-esteem may be critical" (p. 149). Communication skills are basic in psychosocial adaptation, and as such will need to be carefully evaluated and treated to the greatest degree possible.

Prevocational, vocational, and rehabilitation counselors will usually carry the major responsibility for designing prevocational and vocational aspects of the ILP; the social worker usually has major responsibility for planning, implementing, and monitoring the personal-social aspects of the ILP. The psychologist will give input on the cognitive and personality problems and any plans for dealing with them; and the speech/language pathologist and audiologist will both be directly involved in evaluation and intervention with communicative skill problems.

Other disciplines, such as the orthopedic and psychiatric, will provide input by invitation of the team coordinator.

The most common label for the ILP during the early adult years is individualized written rehabilitation plan (IWRP), in accordance with suggestions of the 1978 Rehabilitation Act. Recommended sections of this plan include, among other things, the following minimal information:

1. Physical limitations or medical problems resulting from the client's syndrome.

2. Client skills and deficits in a variety of vocational and enviromental areas and in adaptive behavior.

3. Training opportunities available to the client.

4. Environmental supports available to the client, including social skills training, living arrangements, transportation access, and leisure opportunities.

5. Vocational opportunities. (A.S. Halpern, 1981, p. 274)

The major community resources for cerebral palsied persons in the early adult years are usually funded through the state's adult rehabilitation service administration and to a lesser extent through some phases of the developmental disabilities program.

The logical professional to play the role of team coordinator is the rehabilitation counselor because he or she will likely be most knowledgeable about the availability of appropriate prevocational or vocational training opportunities, which is critical to the development of the IWRP. The rehabilitation counselor is also usually most knowledgeable about potential employment opportunities or employers of the handicapped, and will be the most successful in matching the client up with the most favorable employment context. This knowledge is important because the vocational difficulties of a severely handicapped person are invariably compounded by negative social attitudes of a nondisabled society. "It is important that clients be encouraged to attempt to achieve their maximum potential level of performance by taking occasional risks and sometimes failing and learning from the experience. In general, where suitable alternatives exist, it is preferable for adult clients not to live with their families of origin" (A. S. Halpern, 1981, p. 275). Faced with such frightening circumstances, a severely handicapped client will feel more comfortable having a rehabilitation counselor as an advocate.

Other members of the ILP team, of course, will depend upon the kinds of problems facing the individual and the kinds of training and/or habilitation programs needed.

Communication Problems

Peripheral Sensorimotor Deficits Involved in Communication

If one observes the oral-peripheral speech mechanism in cerebral palsied children whose severity of impairment ranges from moderate to severe in degree, one will observe that there are some rather severe structural as well as functional abnormalities.

Structural deviations are actual deformities observed in the various physical components of the speaking mechanism. Deviations frequently observed in the breathing mechanism include flaring rib cage in the region of the 9th to 12th ribs on either side of the sternum. Deviations often found in the voice mechanism include abnormal position, size, or shape of the larynx (such as unusually high or low position), obtuse thyroid angle created by abnormal muscle pulls on the thyroid cartilage, and an unusually high palate. Deviations often found in the articulation mechanisms include contractures in the tongue and/or mandibular muscles, open bite, and severe dental caries or defective tooth enamel.

Functional deviations are abnormal movements observed in the communication mechanisms during voluntary efforts to speak orally. Functional deviations in the breathing mechanism may include thoracic abdominal opposition or "reversed" breathing, stertorous (or noisy) breathing due to clonic or tonic pharyngeal occlusion, and severe tension in breathing musculature. Abnormal functional deviations may be observed in the vocal mechanisms, which include hyperrhinolalia due to lack of velar closure, respiratory-laryngeal incoordination, spasmodic constriction or dilation of glottis due to overcontraction of laryngeal constrictors or dilators, athetosis of laryngeal musculature, and overflow from arm and shoulder muscles to the vocal mechanisms.

Abnormal functional deviations that may be observed in the articulation mechanism include abnormal deviations of the tongue or soft palate, disjunction of the mandible when it is depressed (mandibular facet slip), lateral deviations of the jaw, inability to elevate the tongue, overt lingual apraxia or inaccuracies of voluntary tongue movement, retraction of the tongue, slow tongue movement, bizarre opening and closing of the lips, involuntary facial movements or grimaces, and drooling.

Hearing impairment has been reported to occur with relatively high incidence in the cerebral palsied population. Severe hearing loss, within the realm of deafness in the legal sense, has been reported to range from 6% to 16% in various studies (Easton & Halpern, 1981). There is a significantly higher incidence of severe hearing loss in kernicterus patients whose cerebral palsy etiology was fetal erythroblastosis, an RH-negative blood incompatability (Hardy, 1961; Lassman, 1951).

Hardy (1961) reported that in a study of 48 kernicterus children, only 9 (18%) demonstrated normal hearing; 26 (52%) were felt to have pure nerve deficit, while 11 (28%) were considered to have higher-level imperception (central auditory processing disorders). Perlstein (1961) reported that 43% of 499 kernicterus children investigated had a hearing loss or hearing imperception. Hearing deficits in the kernicterus group are frequently associated with defective upward (vertical) movement of the eyes (Woods, 1957). (In the past few years, improved fetal diagnoses and treatment have greatly reduced the incidence of kernicterus.)

The sensory and motor neurons in the cranial nerves, which control all aspects of the final common pathway in communication, are not damaged or impaired in the cerebral palsied child. Why then, one may ask, are there so many severe structural and functional muscular and skeletal abnormalities in those who are moderately to severely handicapped?

In order to better understand this apparent contradiction, it is perhaps helpful to consider the evolution of the three-neuron system, which has reached its highest level in the human brain. The one-neuron system is the most primitive form of the evolving nervous system and is illustrated in primitive animals such as sponges (Felton & Felton, 1982). In this nervous system, the neural cell receives stimuli from the environment and initiates movement through stimulation of effector tissues. The main function of this nervous system is to detect noxious stimuli and cause a withdrawal movement.

The two-neuron system evolved to provide for greater diversity of response. In this system, a sensory neuron interacts receptively with the environment, and a separate motor neuron controls the effector tissue. The two-neuron system provides for slightly more discriminating activity in the nervous system, but still only provides for reflexive, all-or-none responses.

In the three-neuron system, the sensory neuron reacts to the environmental stimuli, and an intermediate neuron (interneuron) carries the information to the third neuron, the motor (or effector) neuron. This system allows a graded or partial response and allows responses of the organism to interact with other stimuli being received by the organism. This three-neuron system exists in worms and all other more advanced animals; the interneuron is responsible for differences in information-processing complexities of various organismic hierarchies.

Central Nervous System Relationships

The sensory and motor neurons involved in communication—namely, the cranial nerves—comprise part of what is called the peripheral nervous system (PNS). These nerves have direct contact with the enviroment through sensory receptors or muscle tissue. The interneuron system that handles information processing between the sensory and the motor systems but that does not have direct contact with the outside environment, either through sense organs or muscle tissue, is called the central nervous system (CNS).

Since the cerebral mechanisms are the ones impaired in cerebral palsy, the neuropathology of cerebral palsy is almost exclusively the result of damage to interneurons, which comprise virtually all cerebral mechanisms (Felton & Felton, 1982).

The cranial nerves are the portion of the PNS involved in the reception and production of communication codes. They perform under the control of the interneurons in the CNS. The levels of interneuron control involved depends on the complexity of the behavior being performed.

Segmental spinal reflexes, such as withdrawal of the hand when touching a hot stove, involve only interneurons at or near the segmental level where the reflex occurs. Reflexes involving both flexion and extension movements require a greater number of interneurons and over a broader vertical span in the spinal cord. An example is the crossed extension reflex, which occurs if one steps on a nail; the injured extremity flexes while the extremity on the opposite side extends in order to maintain postural coordination.

More complex reflexes require an even greater number of interneurons spread across a much higher vertical span up the CNS; an example is the tonic labyrinthine reflex, which may involve thousands of interneurons that span vertically from the spinal level up through the brainstem and into the vestibular nervous system.

Voluntary communicative movements involve interneurons at all levels from the medulla up to the cerebral cortex. Therefore, neuromuscular performance for communication could be influenced by neuropathology at any of the various levels that participate in information processing for communication, from the brainstem up through the cerebrum.

In cerebral palsy the motor problem is a lack of control of the muscles rather than muscle weakness. This lack of control is often seen as "a failure of inhibition of some specific central nervous system reflexes" (Easton & Halpern, 1981, p. 137).

Ambulation, balance, and self-help activities such as self-feeding and grooming depend greatly upon finely integrated muscular coordination—i.e., patterns of inhibition and facilitation brought about by coactivation of the alpha and gamma systems. For an excellent discussion of the alpha and gamma systems and their role in facilitation and inhibition, see Darley, Aronson, and Brown (1975). The condition of cerebral palsy, therefore, affects these functions more than any processes involved in the ecosystem. If more than the sensorimotor processing systems are impaired (e.g., cognitive impairment), a child would be considered multiply handicapped and would be labeled cerebral palsied and mentally retarded.

Language Impairments

Table 1 shows a hierarchy of language components, which become progressively more complex and therefore involve a greater number of interneurons as we move up the scale. Furthermore, the higher up the scale in this hierarchy, the less effect specific motor coordination pathology has on their proficiency. Since cerebral palsy is primarily a motor pathology syndrome, the only component maximally devastated by the syndrome is phonological production.

TABLE 1
Model of Language Arranged Hierarchically in Terms of Increasing Complexity

Language Comprehension	Language Production
Pragmatics	Pragmatics
Semantics	Semantics
Grammar	Grammar
Morphology	Morphology
Syntax	Syntax
Phonology	Phonology
Prosody	Prosody
Phonemes	Phonemes

Many cerebral palsied children have multiple handicaps; they have motor incoordination resulting from the cerebral palsy and also have mental retardation as a result of damage to the cognition component in the nervous system. Since the relationship between cognitive pathology and grammar is fairly high and that between cognitive pathology and semantics is even higher, we would expect a severely cognitively impaired child to have severe deficits in higher language functions.

The above relationships have important implications for planning intervention. In the severely cerebral palsied child (i.e., one who has severe motor incoordination of the speech mechanism but little or no impairment of cognition), we would need to work mainly toward improving intelligibility. In a mild cerebral palsied child with severe cognitive impairment, on the other hand, we would need the language pathologist mainly for higher-language facilitation and little or no phonological or intelligibility training.

Dysarthria

Children with cerebral palsy are often difficult to understand because they are limited in flexibility of extent and variety of motor control for proper phonological productions (dysarthria). The phonological deficit may be at the prosodic level involving pitch, stress, and juncture, or at the phonological-process level. Most commonly, a mixture of prosodic and phonological production deficits are present. In a study by Wolfe (1950), 45% of the cerebral palsied children in a representative sample were only partly understandable or were not understood at all. Of this portion of the sample, 40% were rated as being "not understood." The athetoids had the greatest amount of trouble, with 40% being rated as "not understood." Spastics as a group seemed less involved: only 30% of the spastics had speech that was rated partially or totally lacking in understandability. In a study by Lencione (1954) involving a sample of 129 cerebral palsied children in public schools, the athetoids again were found to be much less understandable than the others; 71% of the atheroids had "unintelligible" speech as compared to 31% of the spastics so rated. Ansel, McNeil, Hunker, and Bless (1983) have shown that adult cerebral palsied persons retain a high degree of unintelligibility.

It is relatively easy to recognize that prosodic phonological impairments result mostly from difficulties in rate and variation of movements during spontaneous discourse. This slowing of rate of muscle movement and difficulty getting adequate variation of movement patterns may be found in the breathing and vocal mechanism as well as in the articulating and resonating mechanisms. Difficulties on the prosodic level do not seem to be from lack of knowledge of the phonological stress rules (described by Chomsky & Halle, 1968), but rather lack of inhibition of primitive reflexes during the speaking process, which in turn slow down the rate of movement, impose jerky and/or irregular movement, or impair extent of muscle movement, making it impossible or difficult for various muscle groups to make proper contacts during prosodic and articulatory performance.

Stuttering, or symptoms similar to stuttering, have frequently been reported among the cerebral palsied population. Rutherford (1944) found twice as many "stutterers" in children with cerebral palsy as among other defective speech cases in the Minneapolis public schools. She reported that 54% of the athetoid children had jerky, arrhythmic speech, while 13.15% of the spastics and 7% of the normals exhibited the same kind of speech. Her findings substantiated the contention that the extrapyramidal tract lesions are highly disruptive to the rhythmic functions of speech.

After the first year in infancy in normal children, breathing rate slows down considerably to approximately 20 to 25 breathing cycles per minute. The cerebral palsied child frequently retains very rapid (up to 80 cycles per minute) and irregular breathing for many years (Westlake, 1951). Frequently, abnormalities of the thoracic cage can be observed in a child who appears to have excessive activity of the diaphragm and reduced function in the muscles of the anterior chest wall and neck. It appears, in these cases, that the chest and neck muscles are not capable of maintaining the position of the cage during the time that the diaphragm is active, so that the chest actually sinks during the time of inhalation rather than rising and expanding as it should. The sternum is also often sucked inward in this phenomenon, which Westlake labeled *reversed breathing* (Westlake, 1951). Flattened or flaring rib cages and indented sternums result from abnormal breathing function and muscular imbalance.

Cerebral palsied children vary in their ability to phonate and prolong sounds and sound combinations in speech; their difficulty may be in any or all of the attributes of voice (i.e., pitch, intensity, quality, and variation). Some children are unable to phonate a tone in exciting situations; others have difficulty sustaining a tone for any length of time.

The voice of the athetoid tends to be weak in volume and may have irregular spurts of intense volume in conjunction with involuntary spasms of the diaphragm. The final sounds of words or phrases are often whispered. Monotones are common, and in the extreme tension athetoid, the habitual pitch is often near the upper limit of the voice range.

Intelligibility is not only affected by prosodic phonological disorders, but may also be severely affected (or even devastated) by disordered muscular control involved in the production of phonemes.

In the spastic child, there are several possible types of muscular involvement. The speech musculature may be hypertonic; thus, movement is slow and labored because of the difficulty in getting adequate and smooth reciprocal innervation. Fathergill and Harrington (1949) quote several sources that demonstrate that the muscles of the lower jaw are especially susceptible to the stretch reflex. In reference to some spastics, Phelps (1950) has described the presence of a type of flaccidity, or lack of muscle tone, which he terms *zero cerebral*, or *aspastic spasticity*. In these cases, some of the tongue or jaw muscles may be too weak for adequate movement. There may be overtonicity in some opposing muscles, making synergistic movement difficult.

Frequently these abnormal conditions exist in many muscle groups in the spastic child, and if the tongue and jaw muscles are so involved, the speech of the individual will be greatly impaired. If the extensors of the jaw, for example, are activated to open the jaw, an impulse to the extension muscles will initiate a strong contraction, perhaps a maximal one; the joint will begin movement, and the flexor muscles will be stretched. If the flexor muscles are spastic, they will contract violently as a result of the stretch reflex. Thus, reciprocal action of the jaw is reduced or destroyed (Palmer, 1949). If the child attempts further opening of the jaw, the external pterygoid muscle may contract more strongly and actually pull the condyle forward from its joint (mandibular facet slip).

In athetoid children, the nature of the neuromuscular involvement is different. In this condition, involved muscles suffer from an involuntary movement or series of involuntary movements. If any of the muscles of articulation are involved with athetotic movement, articulate speech may be jerky or arrhythmic and may be accompanied by extra clicks and noises resulting from involuntary movements superimposed on the efforts toward regular movements required in the speaking process. Articulatory problems seem to be present to a much greater degree in the athetoid group than in the other groups of cerebral palsy. The mandibular facet slip and athetosis of the tongue have been frequently observed in the athetoid group (Achilles, 1955; 1956). Abnormal oral-motor reflexes (rooting, etc.) may be present (Mysak, 1963; 1980); and, if so, will further complicate control of fine-motor movements required for speech.

Available reports on articulation are based on clinical observations as well as experimental study. More or less general agreement exists in the literature on the following characteristics of articulation (Irwin, 1972; Van Riper, 1963): (1) tongue-tip sounds and those requiring fine coordination are the most difficult; (2) there are significantly more omissions than substitutions or distortions; (3) movements of the tongue are usually the most difficult of all speech movements; (4) rate of diadochokinesis is generally slow; (5) functional defects are often present instead of or in addition to dysarthria; (6) the difficulty of movement patterns in producing a speech sound is influenced by the patterns of sounds that have come immediately before and those that are to come immediately after; (7) articulation is ineffective (e.g., a sound may be produced in the easiest possible manner), and if it sufficiently serves its purpose, its use is continued even though it might not be the best the person can do; and (8) the final sound positions are, in general, more difficult than initial or medial ones (Irwin, 1972).

Research has not been done on the phonological simplification processes used by cerebral palsied children. Those simplification processes used by normal children in the very early stages of articulation development have been described in the literature (Ingram, 1981). The most frequently used simplification processes include: (1) consonant cluster deletion, in which one or more consonants in a multiconsonant cluster are omitted, with usually only one remaining; (2) stopping, where consonant continuants are replaced by stop-consonants that are produced in the same place; (3) depalatization, in which affricates are depalatalized (e.g., *church* becomes "surs"); (4) fronting, in which back consonants are produced in the same manner but in the front of the mouth rather than in the back (e.g., *koo-koo* becomes "too-too"); (5) gliding, in which liquid consonants are produced as glides (e.g., *red* becomes "wed"); (6) consonant deletion, in which one or more syllables in a word have the consonants deleted (e.g., *top* becomes "ta"). There are a number of other less frequently occurring phonological simplification processes.

Difficulty in neuromotor control in dysarthria may make a number of these processes attractive to cerebral palsied children.

Parents are often said to be able to understand their cerebral palsied children better than other persons less familiar with the child. It is quite probable that parents learn, over a period of exposures to the child's defective speech, what kind of errors or phonological simplification processes a particular child is using and are much more able to "translate" the words than persons not so frequently exposed. This tendency to adapt has some practical implications for treatment and will be discussed further in the next section.

Criteria for Use of a Nonspeech Communication System

Most severely involved and almost all profoundly involved cerebral palsied children have speech production that is virtually impossible to understand because of poor intelligibility or because the child is virtually nonverbal. In spite of this fact, professional workers and parents tend to continue to want to emphasize speech and language training rather than turning to various nonspeech alternative options (McDonald, 1980). McDonald has speculated on one important reason for this inertia:

> It has often been said that speech is "uniquely human." As Denes and Pinson (1963) put it, "Speech, in fact, is one of these few, basic abilities – tool making is another – that set us apart from animals and are closely connected with our

ability to think abstractly." Lieberman and Crelin (1971) suggest that "man is human because he can say so." Not to speak, it is claimed, represents a failure to develop an important human characteristic. Many parents insist that their nonspeaking children be taught to talk. They reject a nonspeech method of expression. Parents, therapists, and children of this persuasion must learn the importance of communication and realize that speech is but one mode of expression. Other channels for expression may be opened when the speech is irremediably disabled. (1980, p. 55)

In 1981, the American Speech-Language-Hearing Association recognized that over 1 million persons in the United States are in need of alternative modes for communication because they cannot speak. In a position paper published in August of 1981, ASHA suggested that the speech/language specialist is the person most likely to be in a favorable position to provide alternative (nonspeech) modes for communication. The October 1981 issue of *Language, Speech, and Hearing Services in Schools* was devoted to nonvocal communication strategies. Also in 1981, the National Student Speech-Language-Hearing Association sponsored a monograph authored by Faith Carlson entitled *Alternative Methods of Communication: A Handbook for Students and Clinicians.* Other publications on nonvocal communication modes appeared and have provided suggestions for deciding the time and circumstances for instituting nonvocal alternative intervention procedures (Schiefelbusch, 1980; Silverman, 1980; Vanderheiden & Grilley, 1976). The following criteria have been gleaned from these various resources, especially as they apply to cerebral palsied clients.

In considering criteria for selection of a nonspeech mode most appropriate for a given child, there are two basic purposes that the nonspeech mode may serve: (1) as an *alternative* for those children who are considered to have a "high-risk" probability of remaining nonspeaking in spite of intensive training; and (2) as an *augmentive* mode for children with a high probability of developing the speech mode and need a nonspeech mode only temporarily.

Children who most likely fall into the first category include those who are congenitally deaf or become deaf prior to development of language; children with severe neuromotor disorders that are accompanied by severe vegetative impairments in those mechanisms involved in speech; and children past 4 years of age whose speech intelligibility is near zero when the content of what is being produced is not cued contextually. For these children the nonspeech mode may be considered an essential substitute for speech.

Children who may not need a nonspeech mode as an alternative to speech but for whom a nonspeech modality of communicating may serve to facilitate more rapid and/or more efficient speech modality include children with a statistically significant discrepancy between cognitive and language development (the cognitive being better); children whose intelligibility is not severely disrupted but could be improved through an augmentive nonspeech mode; children who are severely delayed linguistically and in whom the audiovocal system appears to be weaker than the visual-motor or tactile-motor system.

After the decision is made that a client needs either a nonspeech alternative system or a nonspeech augmentive system, the decision must be further refined by choosing which type of nonspeech system would be most appropriate or feasible, considering a child's strengths and weaknesses. Criteria for fitting a particular nonspeech mode to a particular child must take into consideration cognitive strengths and weaknesses, sensory capacities, and motor capabilities. Prior to making such a decision, a clinician must be aware of the various nonspeech systems available and must know what minimal cognitive, sensory, and motor skills are required for the various systems.

Figure 7 is a taxonomy of communication techniques, symbols, and uses as suggested by ASHA (American Speech and Hearing Association, 1981, August). All of the components of the taxonomy qualify as nonspeech modes except "speech" and "spoken words."

Figure 8 is a modified version of Katz's Survey of Physical Handicap Scale (1954), which shows various types and degrees of physical handicaps likely to be encountered by cerebral palsied children.

Table 2 lists the nonspeech communication system and their various symbol options, along with various deficit combinations that will likely render a system nonfeasible for a child who has those deficits.

Manual signs and/or gestures (ASL, SEE, or Amerind signs) would probably not be feasible for a child who has a moderate to severe visual handicap or a moderate to severe handicap in arm-hand use. Physical boards or charts (pictures, Blissymbolics, Rebus, or Picsyms) would probably not be feasible for a child who has a moderate to severe vision handicap, a severe hearing impairment, or a moderate to severe cognitive deficit. Mechanical typewriters with traditional orthographic symbols would probably not be feasible for a child who has a moderate to severe visual deficit, a moderate to severe handicap in arm-hand use, or a moderate to severe cognitive deficit. Electronic devices and prostheses that use traditional orthography, pictures, Blissymbolics, Rebus, or Picsyms as symbols would probably not be feasible for a child who has a severe visual deficit, a severe hearing deficit, or a severe cognitive deficit.

The next section will discuss various ways for evaluating degree of physical handicap and various language and speech competencies, with special reference to treatment planning and implementation. It will discuss strategies for attempting to bring about improved speech communication and intelligibility and augmentive or alternative nonspeech communication systems, which may be appropriate for a given child.

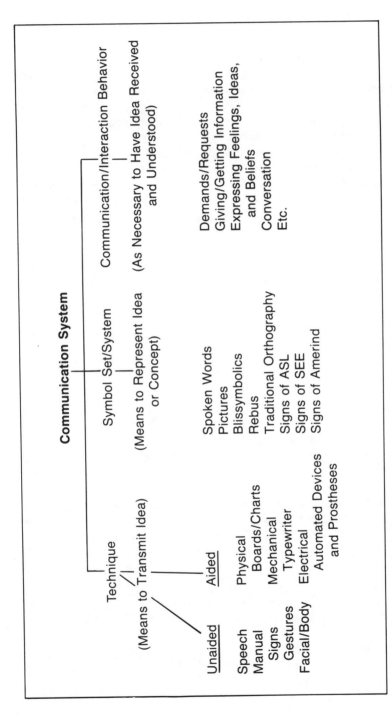

Figure 7. Taxonomy of communication; modes of transmission, alternative symbols, and interaction behavior. From *American Speech and Hearing Association Position Paper* (1981, p. 578). Copyright 1981 by the American Speech-Language-Hearing Association, Rockville, Maryland. Reprinted by permission.

TABLE 2
Taxonomy of Nonspeech Systems and Deficits Affecting Their Feasibility

Nonspeech Systems and Symbol Options	Poor Selection for Children With the Following Deficits
Manual signs and/or gestures; symbol options include: signs of ASL signs of SEE signs of Amerind	Moderate to severe visual deficit Moderate to severe arm-hand use deficit
Physical boards/charts; symbol options include: pictures Blissymbolics Rebus Picsyms	Moderate to severe visual deficit Severe hearing deficit Moderate to severe arm-hand use deficit
Mechanical typewriters; symbol options include: traditional orthography	Moderate to severe visual deficit Moderate to severe arm-hand use deficit Moderate to severe cognitive deficit
Electronic devices and/or prostheses; symbol options include: traditional orthography pictures Blissymbolics Rebus Picsyms	Severe visual deficit Severe hearing deficit Severe cognitive deficit

Assessment

PL 94-142 is called the bill of rights of the handicapped. Under this law, one cannot assume that a child cannot respond to treatment merely upon the basis of symptoms noted. Every child has the right to the most appropriate and least restrictive training program available; every child is given the opportunity to demonstrate whether he or she can respond to treatment strategies, and any lack of progress must be documented by objective data. It operates under the premise that every child can make some progress under appropriate optimal conditions.

The present section therefore not only discusses qualitative procedures for assessing, planning, and implementing treatment, but also attempts to provide suggestions as to how objective assessment, treatment, and generalization data

Survey of Degree of Physical Handicap*

Cerebral Palsy Program, Department of Pediatrics
University of California School of Medicine, San Francisco

Name _____ Sex _____ No. _____ Date _____

Diagnosis _____

Rated by: _____ Date of Birth _____ Age _____

	NON-HANDICAPPING		HANDICAPPING		Comments
	Minimal	*Mild*	*Moderate*	*Severe*	
VISION	☐ No trouble with vision; no glasses needed	☐ Some correction needed; may wear glasses; not handicapped in seeing	☐ Quite handicapped in seeing; vision not correctable by glasses	☐ Almost blind Totally blind	Left eye Right eye
HEARING	☐ No trouble with hearing	☐ Some difficultly in hearing; may wear hearing aid satisfactorily	☐ Quite handicapped in hearing; has difficulty when wearing hearing aid	☐ Almost deaf Totally deaf	Left ear Right ear
SPEECH (verbal)	☐ Speech can be understood without difficulty by a stranger	☐ Some difficulty in being understood by a stranger; able to get ideas across in speech	☐ Speech hard for a stranger or immediate family to understand; hard to get ideas across in speech	☐ Almost totally unable to communicate by speech; totally without speech	

	NON-HANDICAPPING		HANDICAPPING		Comments
	Minimal	*Mild*	*Moderate*	*Severe*	
	☐	☐	☐	☐	
SITTING BALANCE	No difficulty in sitting in a chair or at a table	Somewhat unsteady in sitting in a chair or at a table, but not handicapped in doing so	Quite handicapped in sitting in a chair or at a table; needs a relaxation chair and tray	Unable to maintain sitting balance unless fully supported	
	☐	☐	☐	☐	
ARM-HAND USE	No difficulty in using arms and hands for self-help activity	Some difficulty in using arms and hands for self-help, but not handicapped in doing so	Quite handicapped in using arms and hands for many self-help activities	Unable to use left arm, right arm, arms for any self-help activity	
	☐	☐	☐	☐	
WALKING	No difficulty in walking	Braces needed; unsteady gait; but able to get around	Quite handicapped in walking; cannot walk independently	Unable to walk	Left leg Right leg

*Prepared by Elias Katz, Ph.D., Psychologist, Cerebral Palsy Program, with the cooperation of Dr. Peter Cohen, Associate Professor of Pediatrics and Supervisor of the Cerebral Palsy Program, and staff members.
For method rating, and additional descriptions of behavior for each category, see *Manual*, which can be obtained on request.

Figure 8. Sample of Katz's Survey of Degree of Physical Handicap. From Katz (1954, p. 10) Copyright 1954 by Elias Katz. Reprinted by permission.

can be used to help verify qualititative (subjective) judgments of change over time.

Assessment for treatment will need to provide an estimate of a child's level of communicative competence. This will include an assessment of language developement and use as well as level of speech intelligibility.

In the event the child needs to use a nonspeech augmentive or alternative communication system, assessment needs to provide an estimate of various physical and/or cognitive handicaps and their severity.

The following is an example of an assessment that was made of a 2 1/2-year-old cerebral palsied child whose prospects for developing intelligible communication appeared to be fairly good. As can be seen from the Katz scale (Figure 9), his vision and hearing were within normal limits, his speech was moderately unintelligible (about 40%), his sitting balance was so poor that he was unable to maintain a sitting position unless fully supported, he was unable to use his arms and hands for any self-help activities, and he was completely unable to walk because of severe spasticity in both legs. Cognitive development according to the Piagetian sensorimotor scales appeared to be approximally normal, and language development was only slightly delayed according to the Verbal Language Development Scale. Recommendations for more in-depth assessments were made for the speech pathologist (phonological and intelligibility analyses), the occupational therapist (arm-hand use and self-help feeding, dressing, and grooming skill needs), and the physical therapist (for postural and ambulation skill needs).

The child just described is communicatively more fortunate than the majority of children with severe cerebral palsy; more typically, speech, when existent, is much less intelligible, and the use of an alternative nonspeech substitute would likely be warranted. In this event, arm-hand use usually compensates for severe disability of the speech mechanism. In exploring possible use of a nonspeech alternative mode, assessment of the child's sensory (vision and hearing), motor (hand-arm use), and cognitive skills is extremely important. In the event of severe arm-hand impairment, knowledge of the child's ability to control other parts of the body such as head and eyes becomes important, since these are often used for input control in a number of nonspeech systems.

The Katz scale can serve as a screening procedure for assessment of vision, hearing, arm-hand use, and ambulation. The Katz survey form (see Figure 8) suggests criteria by which one would judge the degree of deficit: minimal, mild, moderate, or severe. Parents or guardians can be extremely helpful in using this survey form for estimating patterns and severity of physical handicap. Such judgments can then serve as a basis for referral to various specialists who can objectively validate the judgments that were made on the basis of the scale and

Cerebral Palsy Evaluation Sheet

Name _____ *Jon Doe* _____ Examiner __ *C. Taker*

Diagnosis _____ *Spastic Quadriplegia* _____

Date Checked _*1983*_ ___*2*___ ___*5*___
               Year   Month   Day

Date of Birth_*1980*_ ___*8*___ ___*7*___ Age _*2 -6*_
            Year   Mondy   Day

Katz—Degree of Physical Handicap

	Minimal	Mild	Moderate	Severe	Comments
Vision	X				
Hearing	X				
Speech			X		
Sitting Balance				X	
Arm-Hand Use				X	
Walking				X	

Social or Mental Maturity: *45%tile* Verbal Language Development *40%tile*

Other Tests: _____ Basal Score: _____

_____ Total Score: _____

_____ Language Age Equivalent: _*1 year*_

Figure 9. Modified form of Katz's Scale of Degree of Physical Handicap for screening a young cerebral palsied child.

who will more than likely be involved in providing appropriate input for the individual habilitation plan.

Verbal language of a young cerebral palsied child is often difficult to assess due to the presence of greatly reduced intelligibility. For this reason, it is usually most feasible to use an informant interview procedure such as the revised Verbal Language Development Scale (Mecham, in press).

Conventional procedures for assessing intelligibility have been described elsewhere (Mecham, 1979; H. Halpern, 1986). An informal method for screening intelligibility and assessing intelligibility changes during intervention is to tape record a 15- or 20-minute segment of spontaneous conversation and have two listeners independently transcribe it without contextual cues. Reliability of the measure can be indexed by noting agreements of the two listeners on the transcriptions; the measure of intelligibility is the percentage of the taped conversation that is correctly transcribed by the listeners. If the child's intelligibility is influenced by context, several samples of spontaneous conversations can be recorded, each in a different context. If changes in intelligibility are to be assessed over time, it is imperative that the samples be recorded in the same contexts and that the same listeners be used for repeated assessment over time.

Competency tests for cognitive skills usually require sophisticated motor movements as responses to be judged; this places a cerebral palsied child at a great disadvantage, since he or she may not be able to respond in such a way as to reveal the actual level of cognition possessed by the child. This same problem interferes with the administration of standard language production tests.

Assessment of such children must rely heavily upon receptive input as the main source of information relative to the child's productive competency. Special modifications in administering such tests as the PPVT-R and BOEHM, which require the child to indicate the correct choice from several choices given, may be made by supplying adaptive equipment such as ETRAM or a head stick, with which the child may indicate his or her selected choice (Carlson, 1981a; Mecham & Willbrand, 1979; Shane, 1980). Such modifications may render exact comparisons of this child's score with the standardized scores for a particular test less accurate, but the information may still be considered to be a more objective estimate of the child's competency than strictly subjective judgments.

Tests of language comprehension probably give a better estimate of a child's language competency than those which tap both comprehension and production or only production; these may need to be modified in such a way that the child can use a method of indicating answers that is within his or her realm of capabilities. Such modifications are sort of a "half-way house" between strictly subjective impressions and highly standardized testing.

Assessment of which nonspeech modality would be best suited to a particular child is not a simple matter. Just as testing in other domains presents problems because of the child's limitations in indicating choices, so testing in the area of nonspeech systems presents many problems. Perhaps the best method is to select the match that looks best according to some preconceived criteria (such as those given in Table 2) and actually give the child a trial period of "diagnostic treatment." Experimental trial periods with a number of alternatives may yield a comparative impression that can be used clinically for decision making (Mecham, 1981).

Treatment Approaches

As McDonald and Chance (1964) observed, "Quite naturally the reader now expects to be told *how* to treat cerebral palsied children. Unfortunately, on this subject there is neither unanimity of opinion nor uniformity of methodology. Many methods for treating cerebral palsied children have been proposed. The strongest supporters of each method are the originators of the method, their students, and those parents whose children seem to have aided by the method .... No scientific evidence available today demonstrates that *one* method of treatment is superior to all other methods. No currently employed system of treating cerebral palsied children has been adequately tested through carefully controlled studies" (pp. 63–64).

Generally speaking, there are two major approaches which are widely used in habilitation of cerebral palsied persons: (1) traditional approaches going back to the early 1950s that stress primarily efforts toward changing the neuromotor skills of the child (neurodevelopmental approaches) and (2) a more current approach that stresses efforts to provide specialized technical equipment and/or facilities to compensate for ineffective neuromotor control (compensatory approach). These two general approaches are not incompatable, but are commonly used conjunctively.

A neurodevelopmental approach is most often used as the major intervention procedure with children who have some intelligible language and good to excellent potential for acquiring accountable changes in neuromotor skills in the areas of communication, self-help, and ambulation. For children with little or no intelligible language and poor or guarded prognosis for neurodevelopmental improvement, the compensatory approach may prove to be most productive, either in conjunction with or in lieu of the neurodevelopmental approach.

Deciding which approach combinations to use must be the responsibility of the multidisciplinary team based upon specific needs and potentials of a given child.

The remainder of this monograph will describe briefly the neurodevelopmental approaches and the compensatory approaches currently in vogue. The reader is cautioned that one cannot become sophisticated in using treatment techniques from such a brief discussion as will be presented here; for this reason, references are given for interested readers who seek much greater detail on both the principles involved and their respective applications. Many of the approaches (e.g., Bobath's approach) require the completion of a special course of training prior to attempting to apply them in treatment.

More detailed general discussions about treatment methods as they apply to communication training can be found in such references as Darley (1962), Hardy (1983), McDonald and Chance (1964), Mecham et al. (1966), Mysak (1980), and Vanderheiden and Grilley (1976). The Mysak reference is especially detailed on the neurodevelopmental approaches, and the Vanderheiden and Grilley reference is especially detailed on the compensatory approaches.

Basic Neurodevelopmental Approaches

The Phelps approach was one of the earliest systems for treatment in the early 1950s. Phelps's method (Phelps, 1950) was aimed primarily at neuromuscular training. He defined several types of muscle conditions: a *spastic* muscle contains too much tonicity due primarily to triggering of the stretch reflex, which is hyperirritable; a *flaccid* muscle (labeled by Phelps as *zero cerebral*) is hypotonic and therefore very weak; an *athetoid* muscle is one afflicted with volleys of unpredictable and arrhythmic and uncontrollable movements. Antigravity muscles seem most prone to have hyperirritable stretch reflexes; athetosis is prone to spread from muscles in proximal (central) areas to other muscles located around more distal (peripheral) joints. Phelps's major approach is bracing, along with intensive training of involved muscles for better control. Muscle training used is the traditional physical therapy approach using such procedures as passive-to-active exercise, a gradual progression from passive to assisted movement, and then through exercise in which assistance is faded out to allow active and voluntary motion to prevail. Two methods are used in implimenting muscle training: (1) resistance (also stressed by other neurodevelopmental authorities) and (2) automatic or "confused" motion, which enables one to capitalize on determining the basic involuntary strength of a muscle and proceed from that level in training. More will be said about "confused" motion later. Relaxation training is an integral part of Phelps's method. Reciprocation is basic for training in ambulation; reach and grasp is basic for other types of self-help development; and skills training in dressing, feeding, toilet care, grooming, and communication serve to functionalize and facilitate improvement in neuromuscular control. Therefore, the core team for the Phelps method includes the teacher, physical therapist, occupational therapist, and speech pathologist.

The Bobath approach was developed by a husband-and-wife team (Bobath & Bobath, 1955) in England. The main objective of the Bobath treatment is to teach control of primitive reflex reactions. This control is attained by a special technique of activating passive movements without permitting abnormal reflex patterns from occurring. These reflex patterns and their uninhibited predominance in cerebral palsy, mentioned in an earlier section, are discussed in greater detail by Bobath (1954) and Capute, Accardo, Vining, Rubenstien, and Harryman (1977). In order to employ the technique, the therapist must have a thorough knowledge of the basic reflex patterns of posture and movement, which normally are inhibited and utilized selectively, as needed, by higher centers of the central nervous system.

The therapist places the child in a posture that is the exact opposite of the one desired by the child. This posture is called a "reflex inhibiting posture" or "rip." Each child has typical postures depending on the site of the lesion, the position of the body in space, and the position of the head and neck in relation to the body. The "rip" for any posture that the child tends to assume involves changing the flexion to extension, pronation to supination, abduction to adduction, etc. These changes are forced by the therapist at the various joints, the proximal joints being the most important (Crickmay, 1955).

In the Bobath therapy, physical therapy and speech therapy go hand in hand. Both physical therapist and speech therapist need special training to enable them to predict reflex behavior and plan appropriate "rips." It is while the child is in a "rip" that the child's neuromotor system assumes a normal state of tonicity; during this momentary period of "normalcy" the child becomes conscious of the influence which the "rip" is having on the neuromotor system and is taught gradually to assume voluntarily these "rips" and the accompanying state of normalcy. As the child is gradually able to achieve a more normal state, neuromotor skills required for normal adaptation are taught.

The Fay approach stresses the utilization of what Fay (1948, 1953) called "muscular reflex therapy." It involves use of phylogenetic patterns of development that are recapitulated in ontogenetic patterns in normal neuromotor development. In treatment, a child is taken through the various patterns of primitive movements, which include moving through three stages of movement patterns in the development of crawling and walking: (1) homolateral (the upper extremity and lower extremity on the same side moving together), (2) homologous (the frog pattern, in which the upper extremities move together and then the lower extremities move together, and (3) crossed-diagonal (the normal pattern of four-legged animals as well as humans). "Passive patterning as the patient is in the prone position is carried out initially; gradually the patient is taught to develop voluntary control over these patterns and to coordinate them into a purposeful response" (Adler, 1975, p. 143).

A method that rejects the notion of single-muscle training and favors facilitation of mass-movement patterns was advocated by Kabat (1952). What distinguishes the Kabat approach from other neurologically oriented therapies is "the focus of its adherents on the means of obtaining maximal excitation of motor units" (Mysak, 1980, p. 147). This approach attempts to achieve maximal activation of a voluntary movement pattern by the use of resistance. Facilitation through resistance is the major focus of this approach, requiring special knowledge on the part of the therapist: "To employ these proprioceptive neuromuscular facilitation techniques in treatment of cerebral palsied patients, a therapist would need to know the mass-movement patterns and their components. It would be essential to know how, where, and when to apply maximum resistance. The therapist must be skilled in employing the appropriate techniques for reinforcing the mass-movement patterns" (McDonald & Chance, 1964, p. 73).

An approach that stresses activation, facilitation, and inhibition of muscle action was introduced by Rood (1954). By activation of sensory receptors through modified sensory stimuli, the synaptic thesholds may be reduced and patterns of movement may be facilitated. Agonist muscles can be facilitated and antagonist muscles can be inhibited through stimulation of the skin receptors and proprioceptive receptors. Athetotic muscles are inhibited by slow brushing (about two times per second or less) across the skin receptors. Spastic muscles can be encouraged in proper agonist-antagonist reciprocation by fast brushing (about five times per second) over the skin receptors. Icing is often used along with brushing and has an enhancement effect over certain muscle groups; it is recommended by some to facilitate the sucking pattern in terms of increased lip and tongue movement (Heiniger & Randolph, 1981, p. 137). Only light-work muscles can be activated by brushing; heavy-work muscles become activated by stretching and resisting. Both stretching and resisting provide proprioceptive input. Stretching is administered to the muscle movement being facilitated and provides a facilitating effect in the proprioceptive receptors. Resistance applied immediately after stretching aids in maximizing the response. Timing and strength of proprioceptive stimulation are very important, and a clinician must become skilled in correct application. Receptors that facilitate mobilizers are given quick, changing stimuli and receptors that facilitate stabilization are given continuous uninterrupted stimuli.

The Rood approach has been elaborated and augmented in recent years; an interested reader may get a better understanding of this rather complicated approach by referring to Farber (1982) and Heiniger and Randolph (1981).

Physiological Approaches for Improving Phonology and Intelligibility

Bloom and Lahey (1978) have represented the components of the communication process as the following model:

> Structure
> Morphology
> Syntax
> Phonology
> Content
> Semantics
> Use
> Pragmatics

Perhaps the portion of the paradigm that has the greatest bearing on speech intelligibility is phonology. For this reason, approaches discussed in the present section all aim at improving the phonological system as the most important avenue for greater intelligibility.

The other components of communication (morphology, syntax, semantics, and pragmatics) will be considered in a later section on compensatory systems, since compensatory systems are highly dependent on nonphonological components of language.

Improvement of intelligibility through a phonological approach is necessarily concerned with a neurophysiological approach because of the great dependency of intelligibility upon the neurophysiological functions of the phonological mechanisms.

Although our present knowledge is still scanty in terms of research in cerebral palsy, we have accumulated enough clinical experience to enable us to custom-design our approach to therapy for each child in terms of the various problems observed during the evaluation process. Since no two children are alike and the complexities of cerebral palsy are variable, it is customary to use various combinations of known approaches and then attempt to adapt techniques to meet the needs of the particular child at any given moment.

The act of speaking is made possible by the movement of muscles in patterns prescribed by the input source of the communication system. The parts that are predominantly involved in the phonological transmission of the coded signal in oral communication are those parts whose primary physiological functions are eating, drinking, breathing, etc. The following discussion will consider some of the procedures that are helpful in obtaining better physiological development of those vegetative processes which usually become impaired during their normal maturation in cerebral palsied children.

Evans (1950) stated many years ago that there are several ways to treat the speech mechanism for cerebral palsy: "First, relaxation; second, relaxation; and third, RELAXATION!" Choiniere (1951) found, in a survey of speech therapies for cerebral palsy, a general agreement that relaxation was the most important aspect of therapy.

Drugs have been used for relaxation with limited degrees of success. The use of drugs has been discussed in detail by Denhoff and Robinault (1960), Keats (1965), and others (Mecham, Berko, & Berko, 1966).

Perlstein (1962) has suggested that one of the best relaxants is being successful in the act. Conversely, continued frustration and lack of success in the performance of the act may serve to increase an already existing drive-tension and may reduce the ease of successful performance.

Stabilization (Phelps, 1950) of the muscles of the neck, shoulders, and trunk has been found to reduce the amount of "overflow" into the speech musculature and may also facilitate voluntary relaxation in this area. The use of stabilization is an especially important phase of the speech training program for the athetoid child. Observation of the motor involvements in the athetoid child will show that an attempted movement in one part of the body will set off disturbances in other parts. For example, movements of the hands may trigger involuntary movement in the face, jaw, tongue, or other speech musculature. Similarly, when one part of the athetoid's body is restrained, a reduction of movement of the other parts results.

The principle involved in stabilization of the speech mechanism is the same principle involved in stabilization of the extremities of the body. Westlake (1951) has suggested various types of stabilization techniques for speech, including a chin strap to control the extensor thrust of the lower jaw as well as sandbags, used with the child lying on his or her back or sitting in a relaxation chair, to stabilize the shoulders and other gross muscle groups that might cause overflow activity into the speech structures. Sometimes stabilization can be achieved by merely holding steady the involved arm of the athetoid child while he or she is concentrating on speaking and controlling the speech muscles. In some cases, stabilization is a forerunner of relaxation. Through it, the child learns to feel a relative state of stability of the immobile muscle groups. The child will then be more able to achieve immobility of muscles voluntarily, through conscious relaxation.

Athetotic tension is somewhat proportional to the amount of emotional stress of a situation. Most older athetoids learn to use certain self-devised methods of stabilization while speaking under emotional stress. One athetoid student in college who enrolled in a fundamental speech course in order to get experience in difficult speaking situations had to rather strenuously hold one hand in the other to reduce the excessive overflow and involuntary movements into his speech musculature while speaking before the class. This procedure facilitated relaxation and tended to minimize facial grimaces and other unnatural movements that created unsatisfactory cosmetic effects. Another athetoid adult, whose arms continually flailed around his head and shoulders, could talk much more easily while sitting on both hands.

Another general technique to be discussed is resistive therapy (Kabat, 1952; Phelps, 1950). Two kinds of results may be achieved through the use of resistive therapy: confusion motion and increased muscular contraction.

Confusion motion is that which occurs in one particular part of the body when another part is moved. It is more likely to occur when the movements of the mobile part are resisted or stopped and the desire to move still continues. Confusion motions have been observed in persons in speech therapy. Some children are more able to close their lips tightly if they bite down hard on a rubber block. Some are more able to close the jaw when this movement is resisted by pulling down on the jaw. A child who could not raise the tip of the tongue voluntarily was able to raise his tongue involuntarily when asked to attempt to push his head back against resistance. Another child's chin was held down as he attempted to close his mouth, and his tongue moved up to the gum ridge.

LeFevre (1952) was able to obtain greater effort on the part of the cerebral palsied child through the use of resistive therapy both for breathing and speech production. According to her, children get better voluntary movement in the process of trying to overcome resistance. This idea evolved from Kabat's method of neuromuscular reeducation through resistance. According to Kabat (1952), resistance increases the facility and summation of excitation in the central motor mechanisms, and this enables a maximal response in voluntary motions.

The effectiveness of confusion and facilitation in actual therapy is not well known. These can be used rather effectively in many cases as aids in the appraisal of movement that is possible in various muscles. For example, if the tongue can be made to rise to the rugae as a result of resistance, the therapist knows that the tongue is able to perform this motion and may feel that the time spent in helping the child to achieve the activity voluntarily is warranted.

The technique of resistance may wisely be used as a last resort in therapy and avoided if easier and more enjoyable techniques are effective in eliciting the desired result. Children usually are not too happy when strong resistance is used about the face and mouth. The effectiveness of this procedure requires a certain amount of insight on the part of the therapist and cooperation on the part of the child.

Clinical experience has shown that speech cannot be normally produced unless there is a normal functioning of the chewing, sucking, and swallowing movements (Rood, 1954). The reverse of this, however, is not always true.

Sometimes there is impairment of voluntary movement even though reflexive movement is still intact (lingual apraxia).

Palmer (1950) has stressed the importance of the chewing, sucking, and swallowing processes in the development of speech in cerebral palsy: "If we assume that the tip of the tongue makes movements in four to six hundredths of a second, and sometimes with even smaller time intervals in this mechanical process of speech, and if we have the tongue unable to manage a bolus of food in five or six minutes, it should be obvious that in order for the speech process to move adequately mechanically, something is going to have to be done about the chewing, sucking and swallowing reflexes" (p. 47). Westlake (1951) used a number of techniques in which he utilized modified feeding activities with the child in a number of different postural positions. Modified nipples are used for very young children as a transition from the bottle to the straw. Even older children may be able to suck a nipple but not a straw, and thus modifying nipples in gradual degrees may finally develop the child's ability to drink from the straw.

In modified feeding, food is first placed on the back of the tongue due to greater success in management there, and then it is gradually placed more toward the front. At first, palatable semiliquids are used and then food of thicker consistency as the child learns to manage it. The postural position varies according to the ability of the child to overcome forces of gravity; from a semi-reclining position at first, the child is moved to an upright one, then to a forward-leaning one, and finally to a prone position.

According to Westlake and Rutherford (1961), in the prone position the essential tongue activity uses the lingual muscles in a similar way to that used in producing consonants; developing the tongue tip elevation is exceedingly important for speech.

The child is placed on his or her stomach on a plinth or other solid surface and is encouraged to propel foods to the back of the throat to be swallowed. A mirror is placed in front of the child so that he or she can see the activity of the masticating structures. If propped up by a pillow under the chest, the child may rest the elbows on the plinth and be able to watch in the mirror without danger of bumping the face. Severely involved children who are beginning this type of activity may have to work gradually from the supine or semisupine postion to the sitting postion, and then to the semiprone and prone positions in handling the foods.

Drooling is one of the most troublesome problems facing speech and occupational therapists, but there is much that can be done about it. Many children do not know that they drool, for their sensory mechanism has not learned to distinguish the feeling of saliva running down over the lower lip and chin. The child should be taught to discriminate, as well as possible, between the feeling of drooling and that of nondrooling by keeping the lips as dry as possible. Drooling should be brought to the child's attention, and he or she should learn to recognize the feel of running saliva. The child should be made conscious of swallowing and should learn to swallow often and should attempt to keep the saliva pushed back to the back part of the mouth, where it can be swallowed. The part played by sensory training in drooling remediation cannot be emphasized enough.

In many instances, feeding the child various kinds of tasty, juicy fruits has been helpful in overcoming drooling in both speech therapy and occupational therapy. The child may watch in the mirror and should be encouraged to attempt to get the juices "down the back door" rather than let them return out the "front door."

Adequate breathing for speech of the cerebral palsied child requires the minimum goal of an even exhalation of at least 10 seconds. The speech therapist should, when possible, share the problem of breathing with the physical therapist, who may directly help the child to establish correct breathing patterns.

Extreme nasal emission, especially if accompanied by insufficient intraoral pressure for proper production of sounds, may be indicative of extreme spastic or flaccid involvement of the palate.

Directional control is an important aspect in breathing for voice and may be accomplished through blowing the breath and prolongation exercises that have been variously described in the literature. This may be especially necessary for the spastic child who usually has difficulty getting the velum up and the mouth open wide enough to prevent hypernasality in speech.

Blowing activities that have been found helpful are blowing a Ping-Pong ball up an inclined plane, blowing plastic bubbles, and blowing on toy wind instruments such as a toy flute. Blowing exercises in group activities will increase motivation through competition for praise and recognition.

J. C. Hardy (1961) and others have reported successful and beneficial results of pharyngeal-flap surgery on cerebral palsied children whose palatal paresis did not seem to respond to nonsurgical treatment. Such surgery may be beneficial in improving intraoral breath pressure in children whose palate is severely disabled but whose tongue and breathing apparatus are not so severely paretic as to make the benefits of such surgery questionable. Increased ability to sustain the voice becomes especially important for cerebral palsied children. As Westlake (1951) has indicated, they should be able to sustain the voice steadily for at least 10 seconds.

Basic to the process of articulation is the ability to open and close the mouth. Even more important is the ability to control the tongue, for it is through the activity of the tongue that the intricate characteristics of speech sounds are produced. The minimum requisite of opening and closing the jaw for speech, as suggested by Westlake (1951), is once per second. Children may show an inclination in therapy to imitate jaw movements of the therapist, other children, or even a mechanical animal such as a duck or dog.

Many cerebral palsied children are prone to hold the mouth in an open position. This may be habitual in some while in others it is pathological. Westlake (1951) describes the "extensor thrust" in which the neuromuscular overflow makes closing the mouth difficult in exciting situations or in any type of voluntary activity. This frequently occurs in the athetoid syndrome and typically involves excessive lowering of the mandible and protrusion of the tongue with the tip extending downward.

Several things may aid the cerebral palsied child who has difficulty in keeping the mouth closed. The child may be periodically reminded to close the mouth if the main trouble is merely remembering to do so. Kinesthetic senses should be sharpened to aid the child in knowing when he or she has the mouth closed or open (Phelps, 1950; Rood, 1954). This may be facilitated by sensory training associated with antidrooling training.

The development of any of the basic skills needed in the mastication process may aid the facilitation of the tongue-elevation skill. Sometimes the child can make the proper movement of the tongue if he or she watches the therapist and imitates the movement. A mirror will be an aid to the child in imitating the therapist.

Hixon and Hardy (1964) suggest that remedial exercises employing speech activities may be much more efficient than those which employ nonspeech movement of these structures. This is based upon their finding that nonspeech movements of the articulators are not closely related to defectiveness of speech.

Tongue-tip movements can sometimes be elicited by placing some applesauce or other palatable food immediately behind the upper teeth with a tongue blade. Peanut butter or a small piece of tape have been effectively used in the roof of the mouth. The child makes vertical movements with the tongue tip in the struggle to remove the substance from the inner gum ridges.

Sometimes, when nothing else works, the tongue may be passively manipulated by the therapist using the fingers or a plastic or metal instrument shaped to fit the tongue. Plastic spoons are not only economical but can also be dipped in hot water and molded to fit various portions of the tongue. Metal instruments are easier to sterilize and can be used over and over again.

Compensatory Approaches to Communication Training

In the last 20 to 30 years, rapid advances in technology have made life considerably easier for the average U.S. citizen, and during the past 10 years, technology for the handicapped has been undergoing a similar explosion. Some of the innovations of importance are as follows: (1) electric wheelchairs, which can be controlled by movements of the tongue, have been a boon for totally paralyzed persons; (2) telecommunication instrumentation and captioned TV programs have aided deaf persons; (3) reading aids have become available for the severely visually impaired; (4) computer implants in the brain to replace the peripheral ear or eye mechanisms are almost past the experimental stage now; (5) artificial bionic limbs have been drastically improved through use of special electrodes that respond to ever-so-slight muscle tensions (made possible through use of a microcomputer); (6) voice synthesizers now on the market provide almost normal communication potential for speechless individuals; and (7) total environmental control systems (ECS) have enabled a totally paralyzed person to control the physical enviroment in the home, transportation, and/or business through the use of special computer interactive switches. These switches are the core of these systems and can be operated in a number of ways—as buttons to be pushed, speech- or breath-sensitive tubes, mouth- or tongue-operated swizzle sticks or pressure gauges, etc. (Silverman, 1980).

The problem with the available technologies is that much is still beyond the reach of the average consumer in terms of cost (Campbell, 1981). The development of the technologies has been sponsored mainly by research money. Marketing the technical devices becomes very risky because the consumer group is relatively small; consumers are not usually well off financially; and government insurance or third-party payments are difficult to secure for purposes of assistance (the certainty of this assistance for any given individual is largely "unknown" and must be evaluated experimentally). The greatest hope is that the cost may eventually be drastically reduced through simplification or improving parts and perhaps recycling. At any rate, rehabilitation services and/or community agencies are in a position to evaluate the appropriateness of an expensive electronic device such as the Handivoice and perhaps even lease equipment to consumers for trial use.

As mentioned earlier, certain nonspeech alternative systems require one profile of skills for their use, while others require different sets. It is the task of the speech-language pathologist or other communicative specialist to decide which nonspeech alternative system best matches the child's repertoire of skills. Table 1 gives a rough approximation of this nonspeech alternative system and motor skills match. In general, children with severe cerebral palsy are not good candidates for manual communication systems but rather respond better to some type of communication board—either mechanical or electronic or both.

Once the nonspeech communication system is decided upon, the clinician will need to work in conjunction with the entire interdisciplinary team in implementing the proposed curriculum of training with the system. Since it is the major communication system for the child, all members of the team should encourage its use.

The following section briefly describes the various nonspeech alternative systems that have proved helpful for cerebral palsied children. The descriptions must be brief, but references are given for the convenience of the reader who seeks more detailed descriptions.

The symbol systems that have been found most useful with cerebral palsied children include concrete objects, pictures, and photographs collected by the child and/or the parent (Carlson, 1981); Picsyms (Carlson, 1981); rebus symbols (Clark & Woodcock, 1976); Blissymbols (McNaughton & Kates, 1980); and English orthography—either typed, printed, or written words and phrases (McDonald, 1980). The specific symbol system will depend upon the child's level of cognitive functioning. (Children at lower levels will need more concrete symbols such as objects or photographs, while children functioning on a higher level may respond well to rebus, Picsyms, or Blissymbols.) A child will not be able to use written or printed symbols until he or she is capable of reading.

The earliest nonspeech communication device used with cerebral palsied children was called a "communication board" by Goldberg and Fenton (1960), and its use has been described by a number of authors (Dixon & Curry, 1973; McDonald, 1980; McDonald & Schultz, 1973). The mechanical communication board is manipulated by hand and is usually in the form of a lap board which fits over the arms of the wheelchair.

Electronic communication boards are operated electronically with some type of switch best suited for operation by the child. Various types of switches that may be used, depending on the needs of the child, are discussed in some detail by Silverman (1980).

Three methods of indicating can be used by the child on a communication board (Harris & Vanderheiden, 1980; Vanderheiden & Grilley, 1976). The first is scanning (including such aids as Roto-Com), in which pictures are placed around in a circle on a clocklike structure whose large hand is rotated mechanically or electronically and can be stopped when it is directly over the picture to be selected. Other types of scanners use scanning lights that can be moved vertically, horizontally, or diagonally and can be stopped at any point in the scanning process; the source of the light can originate internally in the aid itself or can be projected onto the aid from a flashlight mounted on the child's head. A second method is encoding (including such aids as ETRAN), in which code indicators are placed along the horizontal and vertical margins of the board. The point at which a vertical code chosen intersects with a horizontal code chosen is the symbol that the child wishes to convey to the listener. Any of the symbols on the board can be selected by this process in a very similar way that any point on a map can be located by using degrees of longitude and latitude. The third method is direct selection (including such devices as the Auto-Com and the Handivoice). This method requires some means of directly selecting the point on the board, such as pointing to a picture on the board or pressing a particular letter on a typewriter keyboard.

A child may respond better to one of these systems than to another or may progress from one level of indicating (e.g., scanning is the easiest) to another (encoding is more complex).

Language Training

One of the most important considerations in the language acquisition of a severely handicapped child involves what words a child should acquire in the language acquisition process. No other aspect of language development will have a greater impact emotionally or motivationally than the words with which the child works.

Figure 10 presents a worksheet on which a list of words can be evaluated in terms of important motivational criteria suggested by Carlson (1981b). Those words for which the most yesses can be tabulated are the ones most likely to provide the most motivational and functional lexicon. To check to see whether a word belongs to a core list of words, the reader is referred to the core vocabulary list provided in Table 3.

The developmental language curriculum will be approximately the same regardless of whether the child is using a nonspeech system or what type of nonspeech system it is. The author advocates using a system similar to normal child language acquisition procedures; specific modeling and monitoring-assessment techniques have been detailed in a booklet entitled *Modeling Language: A Participation Booklet for Parents* (Mecham & Jones, 1981). This booklet is especially useful in that it is geared primarily to the parent who can serve as a paraprofessional in the intervention process. The parent is able to spend more time with the child (and usually does) than any other member of the interdisciplinary team. Other members of the team should be familiar with the procedures so as to ensure the greatest degree of consistency.

Space will not permit a detailed discussion of helping the cerebral palsied child develop other components of language (i.e., grammar, semantics, and pragmatics). What has been presented in this monograph is information and suggestions that apply specifically to cerebral palsied children and their unique problems.

However, whether the child is using a speech mode or nonspeech mode, he or she will need to develop the various components of language. By and large what is good for language-delayed or language-disordered children will also work well with the cerebral palsied child. Detailed suggestions for language

Word	Within Child's Developmental Level		Within Child's Experience Repertoire		Interesting to Child		Child Comprehends Word		Parent, Teacher, or Close Friends Recommend		Core Word	
	Yes	No	Yes	No	Yes	No	Yes	No	Yes	No	Yes	No

Figure 10. Worksheet for evaluating vocabulary selection for treatment. Words meeting the greatest number of criteria would be the best candidates for selection. Criteria were adapted from Carlson (1981).

TABLE 3
Core Vocabulary

apple	egg	more
	eye(s)	mommy
baby		
ball	fish	no
banana	fix	nose
bang		
bath	get down	off
bear	go	on
bird	gone	owl
boo	good-bye	
book	good girl (boy)	pants
bread		phone
brush	hair	play
bubble	hat	
burn	hello	sh
bus	hot	shoe
button		sick
bye-bye	it	sleep
		sock
candy	juice	spoon
car		sweets
cat	key	
clock	kick	Teddy
coat	kitty	there
cookie		today
	lamb	toe
Daddy	light	tomorrow
dinner	lion	tree
dog	look	
door	love	water
down		
drink	milk	yes
	mine	
ear		
eat		

Sources: Gillham (1979, pp. 69–74) and Nelson (1973, pp. 1–135).

therapy are offered by Aram and Nation (1982), Bloom and Lahey (1978), and Mecham and Willbrand (1985). Additional references can be gleaned from these sources if the reader is inclined to pursue further therapeutic techniques in the area of language disorders.

References

Achilles, R. F. (1955). Communicative anomalies of individuals with cerebral palsy: I. *Cerebral Palsy Review, 16*, 15–24, 27.

Achilles, R. F. (1956). Communication anomalies of individuals with cerebral palsy: II. *Cerebral Palsy Review, 17*, 19–26.

Adler, S. (1975). *The non-verbal child.* Springfield, IL: Charles C. Thomas.

American Speech and Hearing Association position paper. (1981). *ASHA, 23* (8), 578.

Ansel, B. M., McNeil, M. R., Hunker, J. C., & Bless, D. M. (1983). The frequency of verbal acoustic adjustments used by cerebral palsied–dysarthric adults when faced with communicative failure. In W. R. Berry (Ed.), *Clinical dysarthria* (pp. 85–108). San Diego: College-Hill Press.

Aram, D. M., & Nation, J. E. (1982). *Child language disorders.* St. Louis: C. V. Mosby.

Batshaw, M. L., & Perret, Y. M. (1981). *Children with handicaps: A medical primer.* Baltimore: Paul Brooks.

Berko, F. G., Berko, M. J., & Thompson, S. C. (1970). *Management of brain-damaged children.* Springfield, IL: Charles C. Thomas.

Bloom, L., & Lahey, M. (1978). *Language development and language disorders.* New York: John Wiley & Sons.

Bobath, B. (1954). A study of abnormal postural reflex activity in patients with lesions in the central nervous system. *Physiotherapy, 40*, 259–373.

Bobath, K., & Bobath, B. (1955). Tonic neck reflexes and righting reflexes in the diagnosis and assessment of cerebral palsy. *Cerebral Palsy Review, 16*, 4–26.

Campbell, J. (1981). New technologies: Dramatic advances for disabled persons. *Disabled USA. 16.* 16–19.

Capute, A. J., Accardo, P. I., Vining, E. P. G., Rubenstein, J. E., & Harryman, S. (1977). *Primitive reflex profile.* Rockville, MD: Aspen Systems.

Cardwell, V. E. (1956). *Cerebral palsy – advances in understanding and care.* New York: Association for Aid of Crippled Children.

Carlson, F. (1981a). *Alternative methods of communication: A handbook for students and clinicians.* Danville, IL: Interstate Printers and Publishers.

Carlson, F. (1981). A format for selecting vocabulary for the nonspeaking child. *Language, Speech, and Hearing Services in Schools, 12*, 240–245.

Choiniere, R. L. (1951). A survey of therapies for the cerebral palsied. *Speech Monographs, 18*, 238.

Chomsky, N., & Halle, M. (1968) *The sound pattern of English.* New York: Harper & Row.

Clark, C. R., & Woodcock, R. W. (1976). Graphic systems of communication. In L. Lloyd (Ed.), *Communication assessment and intervention strategies* (pp. 549–606). Austin, TX: PRO-ED.

Courville, C. B. (1954). *Cerebral palsy.* Los Angeles: San Lucas Press.

Crickmay, M. (1955). *Description and orientation of the Bobath method with reference to speech rehabilitation in cerebral palsy.* Chicago: National Society for Crippled Children and Adults, Inc.

Cruickshank, W. M., & Bice, H. V. (1955). Personality characteristics. In W. M. Cruickshank & G. M. Raus (Eds.), *Cerebral palsy* (pp. 115–165). New York: Syracuse University Press.

Cruickshank, W. M., & Dolphin, J. E. (1951). The educational implications of psychological studies of cerebral palsied children. *Journal of Exceptional Children, 18,* 1–8.

Darley, F. A. (Ed.). (1962). *Symposium on cerebral palsy.* Washington, DC: American Speech and Hearing Association.

Darly, F. L., Aronson, A., & Brown, J. R. (1975). *Motor speech disorders.* Philadelphia: W. B. Saunders.

Denes, P. B., & Pinson, E. N. (1963). *The speech chain.* Baltimore: Williams & Wilkins.

Denhoff, E., & Robinault, I. P. (1960). *Cerebral palsy and related disorders.* New York: McGraw-Hill.

Dixon, C. C., & Curry, B. (1973). Some thoughts on the communication board. *Journal of Speech and Hearing Disorders, 38,* 73–88.

Easton, J. K. M., & Halpern, D. (1981). Cerebral palsy. In W. C. Stolov & M. R. Clowers (Eds.), *Handbook of severe disability.* Washington, DC: U.S. Government Printing Office.

Evans, M. F. (1950). Children with cerebral palsy. In W. Johnson (Ed.), *Speech problems in children* (pp. 158–189). New York: Grune & Stratton.

Farber, S. D. (1982). *Neurorehabilitation: A multisensory approach.* Philadelphia: W. B. Saunders.

Fathergill, P., & Harrington, R. (1949). The clinical significance of the stretch reflex in speech reeducation for the spastic. *Journal of Speech and Hearing Disorders, 14,* 353–355.

Fay, T. (1948). The neurophysical aspects of therapy in cerebral palsy. *Archives of Physical Medicine, 29,* 327–334.

Fay, T. (1953). Desperately needed research in cerebral palsy. *Cerebral Palsy Review, 14,* 11, 13, 15.

Felton, D. L., & Felton, S. (1982). A regional and systemic overview of functional neuroanatomy. In S. D. Farber (Ed.), *Neurorehabilitation: A Multisensory approach* (pp. 1–106). Philadelphia: W. B. Saunders.

Finnie, N. R. (1968). *Handling the young cerebral palsied child at home.* New York: E. P. Dutton.

Gillham, B. (1979). *The first words programme.* Austin, TX: PRO-ED.

Glick, S. J. (1953a). Emotional problems of 200 cerebral palsied adults. *Cerebral Palsy Review, 14,* 3–5.

Glick, S. J. (1953b). Facing an unsolved problem: Employment of the cerebral palsied. *Journal of Rehabilitation, 19,* 7–9.

Goldberg, H. R., & Fenton, J. (1960). *Aphonic communication for those with cerebral palsy: Guide for the development and use of a communication board.* New York: United Cerebral Palsy of New York State.

Halpern, A. S. (1981). Mental retardation. In W. C. Stolov & M. R. Clowers (Eds.), *Handbook of severe disability* (pp. 265–278). Washington, DC: U.S. Government Printing Office.

Halpern, H. (1986). *Language and motor speech disorders in adults.* Austin, TX: PRO-ED.

Hardy, J. C. (1961). Surgical management of palatal paresis and speech problems in cerebral palsy. *Journal of Speech and Hearing Disorders, 26,* 320–325.

Hardy, W. G. (1961). Auditory deficits in the kernitcterus child. In C. A. Swinyard (Ed.), *Kernicterus in cerebral palsy* (pp.255–266). Springfield, IL: Charles C. Thomas.

Hardy, W. G. (1983). *Cerebral palsy.* Englewood Cliffs, NJ: Prentice-Hall.

Harris, D., & Vanderheiden, G. C. (1980). Enhancing the development of communication interaction. In R. L. Schiefelbush (Ed.), *Nonspeech language and communication: Analysis and intervention* (pp. 227–258). Austin, TX: PRO-ED.

Heiniger, M. C., & Randolf, S. L. (1981). *Neurophysiological concepts in human behavior.* St. Louis: C. V. Mosby.

Hixon, T. J., & Hardy, J. C. (1964). Restricted motility of the speech articulators in cerebral palsy. *Journal of Speech and Hearing Disorders, 29,* 293–306.

Hohman, L. B., & Freedheim, D. K. (1958). Further studies on intelligence levels in cerebral palsied children. *American Journal of Physical Medicine, 37,* 90–97.

Hopkins, T. W., Bice, H. V., & Colton, K. G. (1954). *Evaluation and education of the cerebral palsied child.* Washington, DC: International Council for Exceptional Children.

Ingram, D. (1981). *Procedures for the phonological analysis of children's language.* Austin, TX: PRO-ED.

Irwin, O. C. (1972). *Communication variables of cerebral palsied and mentally retarded children.* Springfield, IL: Charles C. Thomas.

Kabat, H. (1952). Central facilitation: The basis for treatment of paralysis. *Permanente Foundation Medical Bulletin, 10,* 190–204.

Katz, E. (1954). A "survey of degree of physical handicap." *Cerebral Palsy Review, 15,* 10–11.

Keats, S. (1965). *Cerebral palsy.* Springfield, IL: Charles C. Thomas.

Lassman, F. M. (1951). Clinical investigation of some hearing deficiencies and possible etiological factors in a group of cerebral palsied individuals. *Speech Monographs, 18,* 130–131.

LeFevre, M. C. (1952) A rationale for resistive therapy in speech training for the cerebral palsied. *Journal of Exceptional Children, 19,* 61–64.

Lencione, R. M. (1954). A study of the speech sound ability and intelligibility status of a group of educable cerebral palsy children. *Speech Monographs, 21,* 213–214.

Lieberman, P., & Crelin, E. S. (1971). The speech of Neanderthal man. *Linguistic Inquiry, 2,* 203–222.

McDonald, E. T. (1976). Design and application of communication boards. In G. C. Vanderheiden & K. Grilley (Eds.), *Non-vocal communication techniques and aids for the severely physically handicapped* (pp. 105–119). Austin, TX: PRO-ED.

McDonald, E. T. (1980). Early identification and treatment of children at risk for speech development. In R. L. Schiefelbusch (Ed.), *Nonspeech language and communication: Analysis and intervention* (pp. 49–80). Austin, TX: PRO-ED.

McDonald, E. T., & Chance, B., Jr. (1964). *Cerebral palsy.* Englewood Cliffs, NJ: Prentice-Hall.

McDonald, E. T., & Schultz, A. R. (1973). Communication boards for cerebral palsy children. *Journal of Speech and Hearing Disorders, 38,* 73–88.

McNaughton, S., & Kates, B. (1980). The application of Blissymbolics. In R. L. Schifelbusch (Ed.), *Nonspeech language and communication: Analysis and intervention* (pp. 303–322). Austin, TX: PRO-ED.

Mecham, M. J. (1954). Complexities in the communication of the cerebral palsied. *Cerebral Palsy Review, 15,* 9–11, 14.

Mecham, M. J. (1979). Cerebral palsy and other neurogenic dysarthrias. In B. V. Hutchinson, M. L. Hanson, & M. J. Mecham (Eds.), *Diagnostic handbook of speech pathology* (pp. 277–294). Baltimore: Williams & Wilkins.

Mecham, M. J. (1981). Analysis and measurement of changes in normal and disordered speech and language behavior. In N. J. Lass (Ed.), *Speech and language: Advances in basic research and practice* (Vol. 5, pp. 80–153). New York: Academic Press.

Mecham, M. J. (in press). *Verbal language development scale – revised.* Salt Lake City: Communication Research Associates.

Mecham, M. J., Berko, M. J., & Berko, F. G. (1960). *Speech therapy in cerebral palsy.* Springfield, IL: Charles C. Thomas.

Mecham, M. J., Berko, M. J., & Berko, F. G. (1966). *Communication training in childhood brain damage.* Springfield, IL: Charles C. Thomas.

Mecham, M. J., & Jones, J. D. (1981). *Modeling language: A participation booklet for parents.* Salt Lake City: Communication Research Associates.

Mecham, M. J., & Willbrand, M. L. (1979). *Language disorders in children.* Springfield, IL: Charles C. Thomas.

Mecham, M. J., & Willbrand, M. L. (1985). *Approaches to treatment of language disorders in children.* Springfield, IL: Charles C. Thomas.

Mysak, E. D. (1963). *Reflex therapy in treatment of cerebral palsy.* New York: Teachers College, Columbia University Press.

Mysak, E. D. (1980). *Neurospeech therapy for the cerebral palsied* (3rd ed.). New York: Teachers College, Columbia University Press.

Nelson, K. (1973). Structures and strategy in learing to talk. *Monographs of the Society for Research in Child Development, 38,* (No. 149).

O'Reilly, D. E. (1975). Care of the cerebral palsied: Outcome of the past and needs of the future. *Developmental Medicine and Child Neurology, 17,* 141.

Palmer, M. F. (1949). Speech disorders in cerebral palsy. *Nervous Child, 8,* 193–292.

Palmer, M. F. (1950). Speech disorders in cerebral palsy. In M. Abbott (Ed.), *Proceedings of the Cerebral Palsy Institute.* New York: Association for Aid of Crippled Children, Inc.

Perstein, M. A. (1961). The clinical syndrome of kernicterus. In C. A. Swinyard (Ed.), *Kernicterus in cerebral palsy* (pp. 268–279). Springfield, IL: Charles C. Thomas.

Perstein, M. A. (1962). Principles of therapy. In F. L. Darley (Ed.), *Symposium on cerebral palsy* (pp. 30–36). Washington, DC: American Speech and Hearing Association.

Phelps, W. M. (1950). Etiology and diagnostic classification of cerebral palsy. In M. Abbott (Ed.), *Proceedings of the Cerebral Palsy Institute* (pp. 1–19). New York: Association for Aid of Crippled Children, Inc.

Rood, M. S. (1954). Neurophysiological reactions as a basis for physical therapy. *Physical Therapy Review, 34,* 444–448.

Rutherford, B. R. (1944). A comparative study of loudness, pitch, rate, rhythm, and quality in the speech of children handicapped by cerebral palsy. *Journal of Speech and Hearing Disorders, 9,* 213–271.

Schiefelbusch, R. L. (Ed.). (1980). *Nonspeech language and communication: Analysis and intervention.* Austin, TX: PRO-ED.

Shane, H. C. (1980). Approaches to assessing the communication of non-oral persons. In R. L. Schiefelbush (Ed.), *Nonspeech language and communication: Analysis and intervention* (pp. 197–224). Austin, TX: PRO-ED.

Silverman, F. H. (1980). *Communication for the speechless.* Englewood Cliffs, NJ: Prentice-Hall.

Vanderheiden, G. C., & Grilley, K. (1976). *Non-vocal communication techniques and aids for the severely handicapped.* Austin, TX: PRO-ED.

Uzgiris, I., & Hunt, J. McV. (1975). *Assessment in infancy.* Urbana: University of Illinois Press.

VanRiper, C. (1963). *Speech correction, principles and methods.* Englewood Cliffs, NJ: Prentice-Hall.

Westlake, H. (1951). Muscle training for cerebral palsied speech cases. *Journal of Speech and Hearing Disorders, 16,* 103–109.

Westlake, H., & Rutherford, D. *Speech therapy for the cerebral palsied.* Chicago: National Society for Crippled Children and Adults, Inc.

Wolfe, W. G. (1950). A comprehensive evaluation of fifty cases of cerebral palsy. *Journal of Speech and Hearing Disorders, 15,* 234–251.

Woods, G. E. (1957). *Cerbral palsy in childhood.* Bristol: John Wright & Sons.

Merlin J. Mecham is a Professor in the Department of Speech Pathology and Audiology at the University of Utah. He has published numerous articles and two previous books on cerebral palsy. He has served as editorial consultant to the *Journal of Speech and Hearing Disorders*, is a member of the editorial board of *Topics in Language Disorders*, and has authored several books and chapters on language disorders. His tests on language development and audiolinguistic processing have been widely used both nationally and internationally. He is a member with licensure in speech pathology and a past president of the Utah Speech and Hearing Association. He is a member with certification in speech pathology, a member of the Congressional Action Committee, a former site visitor for the Educational Training Board, and a satellite instructor on problems in aging for the American Speech-Language-Hearing Association. He is also a Fellow in the association.